WHEN **CANCER** ENTERED OUR FAMILY

WHEN **CANCER** ENTERED OUR FAMILY

How we lived, laughed, cried and survived

Moyra McDill

NOVALIS

© 2007 Novalis, Saint Paul University, Ottawa, Canada

Cover design and layout: Pascale Turmel
Cover image: Glebe Photo (photographer unknown)

Interior photographs by Moyra McDill or Alan Oddy, except for the following: Leonard Oddy (pp. 14, 61, 199); Lars-Erik Lindgren (p. 140); Peter Frise (p. 242); Robert Langlois (p. 267); John Hayes (p. 270); Sarah Oddy (p. 277).

Interior illustration: Linda Cook (p. 224)

Business Offices:

Novalis Publishing Inc.
10 Lower Spadina Avenue, Suite 400
Toronto, Ontario, Canada
M5V 2Z2

Novalis Publishing Inc.
4475 Frontenac Street
Montréal, Québec, Canada
H2H 2S2

Phone: 1-800-387-7164
Fax: 1-800-204-4140
E-mail: books@novalis.ca
www.novalis.ca

Library and Archives Canada Cataloguing in Publication

McDill, Moyra
    When cancer entered our family : how we lived, laughed, cried and survived / Moyra McDill.

ISBN-13: 978-2-89507-835-7
ISBN-10: 2-89507-835-1

    1. Oddy, Alan Sinclair, 1956–. 2. McDill, Moyra, 1956–. 3. Cancer–Patients–Biography. 4. Cancer–Patients–Family relationships. I. Title.

RC265.6.O33M23 2007   362.196′9940092   C2006-906316-8

Printed in Canada.

We acknowledge the financial support of the Government of Canada through the Book Publishing Industry Development Program (BPIDP) for our publishing activities.

5   4   3   2   1   11   10   09   08   07

Lovingly dedicated

to

Leonard (1923–2005) and Lorna, Alan's parents,

and to

Sarah, Andrew and Carolyn, our children

CONTENTS

FOREWORD

At some point in time, every family faces a crisis, in one form or another. And when that crisis occurs, everything changes. Crisis destabilizes. It shakes us up, and we can never return to the way we once were. Every family will deal with a crisis in their own way, according to their combined strengths and vulnerabilities.

In her award-winning novel *A Complicated Kindness*, Miriam Toews writes about Nomi, a teenage girl trying to come to grips with a crisis in her family. Towards the end of the book, Nomi says, "It's hard to grieve in a town where everything that happens is God's will. It's hard to know what to do with your emptiness when you're not supposed to have emptiness."

Moyra McDill, in chronicling how her family lived with the many consequences of her husband's cancer, has created a space where we can experience the emptiness that a serious illness brings to our lives. With honesty and great courage, Moyra and Alan chose to enter the "emptiness" created by his cancer diagnosis. In the process, they discovered much about themselves and about the values and beliefs that shaped their lives.

As dedicated scientists and researchers at heart, they chose a difficult route, continually seeking out the latest and best possible treatments to fight Alan's brain tumour. However, pursuing a cure for Alan wasn't only about their own family's needs and concerns. It would have been much easier, at several points along the way, to stop fighting. But time and again, they decided to keep searching for another drug, another treatment, in the hope that Alan's experience would help other cancer patients and their families. Their determination, and Moyra's decision to document their journey through this unknown territory, is remarkable. I am convinced that their efforts have advanced the knowledge of the medical world, improving the quality of life for many people who face a similar struggle.

While Alan had to come to terms with the limitations of his illness and the possibility of his own death, Moyra was facing a very different reality. Her future now held the possibility of living without the man she loved, the man whom she'd married and with whom she'd had children, the man with whom she had hoped to grow old. In addition to keeping her career afloat and attending to Alan's ever-increasing physical and emotional needs, Moyra also had to care for the needs of their three young children, with all their fears, questions and concerns. As well, she kept in touch with the many family members, friends and colleagues who wanted to support her family through this harrowing time, and who had their own fears and sadness to deal with.

Despite her heavy load of responsibilities and the constant demands on her time and inner resources, Moyra recorded and reflected on all that the family was experiencing. She wrote e-mails on a regular basis to let people know what was happening and how the family was doing, and as you will see, she did so with clarity, humour and grace.

Moyra's writing reflects her profound love for and commitment to her family. She draws the reader into their story, yet never asks for pity. She approaches the all-too-frequent mishaps and setbacks with unrelenting energy and an optimism that is always grounded in reality.

After reading this book, I feel that I have come to know Alan. He moves through his cancer treatments and towards an unknown future in the same way that he lived – with a no-nonsense and wickedly funny take on life. While he rejected an institutional image of God, he wrestles with the big questions of life and meaning in a way that makes sense to him. I appreciate how Moyra accepts and honours his system of belief while remaining true to her own relationship with God and the church. Her attitude speaks volumes for their respect for each other.

Moyra has done a great service in writing this book. Her personal journey – from the diagnosis through countless tests, treatments and beyond – will help anyone who is supporting a friend or family member who has a life-threatening illness. Moyra's story provides key insights to help people struggling to understand what might be happening behind the medical facts and statistics. With her, the reader walks through one of the most heart-breaking experiences imaginable, and discovers that life is stronger than death – but not always in the ways that we might hope or wish for.

While there are many ways to deal with a crisis when it occurs, there is no right or wrong way. What works for one family may not work for another. As we see in this book, Moyra and Alan approach life in a scientific manner – observing, analyzing and solving any challenges that come their way. Faced with Alan's diagnosis, they respond by doing what they know best: they question and research, they document and cross-reference their findings, pushing at the limits of what is known about this form of cancer.

Moyra writes that she and Alan are pursuing every treatment possible because, ultimately, they want to choose life. I believe they did just that. Within the seeming emptiness that the diagnosis of cancer heralded, they encountered fullness – a fullness of love and compassion, poured out from far and wide.

Moyra's book offers the reader an opportunity to discover new perspectives on his or her own experience. The similarities between Moyra's story and mine, for example, are uncanny. My husband, Jean-Marc, was diagnosed at age 35 with the same kind of tumour as Alan's. We, too, had three young children (ours were all under the age of five). Like Moyra and Alan, we were in the building stage of our lives, both professionally and personally. A serious illness like cancer just wasn't part of our plans.

The diagnosis of a grade 4 brain tumour – especially in a young and healthy person – is literally beyond belief. I identified strongly with the shock, numbness and fear that Moyra describes at Alan's initial diagnosis. The tumour was real, very real, and it wasn't about to go away soon. As I read Moyra and Alan's story, I felt I was reading my own family's story. My experience of living with and beyond my husband's cancer is similar in many ways, yet it is different.

In the same way, your story of living with a challenging situation is probably similar, but different. How important it is that we share our stories with one another, for it is in the telling and the listening that we grow and are strengthened. In our time of need we come to know that we are supported, even carried, by the love and concern of family, friends, even strangers. In the community of caring that is created, there is space to experience emptiness, to grieve, and to begin the journey of healing.

Caryl Green
Chelsea, Quebec

PROLOGUE

There he was, leaning against his locker, sporting a hair-out-to-there look, talking to a friend and wearing chain mail mittens! I was more than a little curious as to why one of my engineering classmates would be wearing chain mail. So, while I had spoken to Alan Oddy several times before, and on one occasion he had even informed me somewhat smugly that he had scored more than 100 per cent in a calculus test, it was the chain mail mittens that inspired me to stop and talk. I was intrigued that anyone would have such a thing, and even more so that he had made them himself by winding bits of copper wire to make the rings and then hooking the rings together to make the mittens. We became friends immediately and laboratory partners shortly after.

One winter night, while working on our respective computer programming assignments, Alan and I opted to run between buildings rather than take the long walk through the tunnels under Carleton University. I slipped on the ice and broke my right foot. Our first real date was the end-of-year banquet a few weeks later. I wore a long dress and a cast. We fell in love and, very romantically, became secretly engaged and remained that way until we made a formal announcement at Christmas of our third year. We were married by the Anglican tradition of reading the banns in my little parish church, St. James, in 1978, just before fourth year. At one of the summer services we attended as part of the reading of the banns, the priest began, "We have good news today from St. John." Alan apparently thought of Saint John, New Brunswick – not the saint named John, which confirmed my suspicions that the man I was soon to marry was not overly familiar with the liturgy.

Our lives together took us through our master's degrees, jobs in Halifax and Niagara Falls, and doctorates back at Carleton University. I began my new career as an assistant professor at Carleton and Alan became a post-doctoral fellow at a government laboratory.

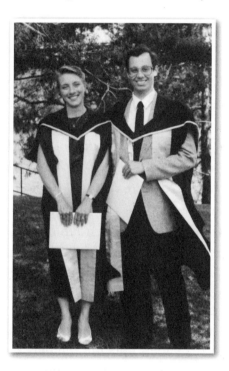

FRESHLY MINTED DOCTORATES, CARLETON UNIVERSITY, CLASS OF 1988.

We were blessed with the arrival of our daughter Sarah in 1989, and twins, Andrew and Carolyn, in 1994. By this point, I had tenure in the faculty of engineering and Alan, who had been a research associate at the government lab and, later, at Carleton, had started a consulting business in numerical analysis.

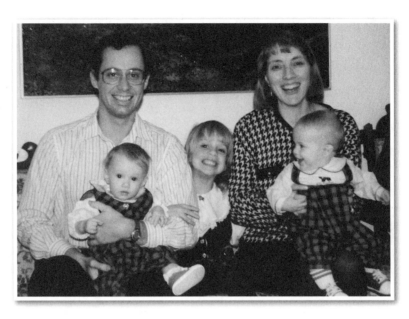

ALAN HOLDING CAROLYN, SARAH, MOYRA HOLDING ANDREW.

As with many married couples, we had our ups and downs, moments of joy and times of sadness. Alan struggled with depression for a decade or more but, by 1996, he had achieved a level of happiness that he had not felt for many years. Still, as the months before our 20th anniversary approached, I was uneasy: he often seemed tired and angry, and he was making little mistakes. At the same time, he was doing some of the most intellectually challenging work of his life, and it was outstanding. It was easy to attribute his difficulties to increased stress from his business, combined with his life as the father of three children. Otherwise, things were going very well. My promotion to full professor had come through and my research was coming along nicely. Alan's business was a going concern and the children were healthy, busy little people.

August 1998 began with twin cases of chicken pox. Carolyn was still quite spotty when Alan had surgery to deal with his snoring, a combined tonsillectomy and uvuloplasty (the removal of the uvula at the back of the throat). We had put the surgery off for several years, but when Andrew wandered into our bedroom complaining that a truck was driving through his room over and over, Alan agreed it was time. He sent this e-mail to a friend.

Sunday, August 9, 1998 – Alan, who had just turned 42, to Peter, recovering from knee surgery

Thanks for the birthday wishes. I hope you are on your feet again as soon as possible. To celebrate my birthday I have decided to have my tonsils removed. I go in Wednesday, also under general anesthetic. We old guys are starting to fall apart. I'm having my tonsils out in the hopes my snoring will be reduced. Andrew has been complaining that the truck in his bedroom is scaring him at night. Moyra says either the doctor does it or she will, with a brick! Personally, I think her sleep problems come from a troubled conscience. I sleep just fine.

Alan

Alan should have recovered easily from his surgery, but he did not. He had terrible headaches several times a day and referred to "the fog rolling in" when he tried to work. At first, the surgeon thought it might be a reaction to the general anesthetic. During a later call to our family doctor, she suggested a secondary infection, so we visited the local hospital emergency room, where Alan was given antibiotics. It turned out that the headaches were far more significant than we could have imagined.

On August 26, 1998, Alan and I celebrated our 20th anniversary. The next morning, Alan was in the tiny ensuite bathroom off our bedroom when he had two massive seizures. I heard the first from the other bathroom. I thought the kids were playing roughly on the rocking chair in our room and making it bounce. A few minutes later, I heard the second one start. I went to check, only to find Alan on the ground, kicking the bathroom walls in a steady cadence. Then it was over – except he was not breathing and there was blood all over the floor. I assumed his throat was hemorrhaging. Sarah called 911 while I rolled Alan on his side, expecting to have to clear his airway of blood. He started to breathe in a horrible, raspy pattern through his clenched teeth. I later learned he had bitten his tongue several times during the seizures.

The firefighters arrived first and put Alan on oxygen. The ambulance came soon after. By then, Alan was coming around, clearly unresponsive on one side. I had the children kiss him goodbye and he left. I followed shortly after when his parents arrived to care for the children.

At the hospital, Alan was undergoing tests, including a CT (computerized tomography) scan. As I sat in the emergency room, I was convinced that the weakness on his left side was the result of a stroke. Knowing that certain drugs had to be given within a few hours of a stroke, I was concerned. When I approached the resident, all she could say was, "I'm so sorry." When I asked again just what was wrong, she said they thought it was a glioma of some kind. From my distant high school biology, I knew we were talking glial cells – brain cells – and the bottom dropped out of my life.

Time began to move very slowly. I remember the resident again saying, "I'm so sorry." I remember that she said it was her first day on that rotation. I remember Alan's parents coming to emergency to support us. I remember Alan laughing and saying he was going to be fine. I remember a doctor offering the glimmer of hope that it was merely a serious brain infection caused by his earlier surgery. I remember going home and vomiting over and over as my body reacted violently to the news, and I remember calling the office to say I wouldn't be in for a few days.

1

August to December 1998
DIAGNOSIS AND RADIATION

Thursday, August 27, 1998 – from an office colleague to friends

Moyra has just phoned to tell me that Alan has been diagnosed today with a brain tumour the size of a golf ball on his brain. It is too early for a full diagnosis, but obviously the news is bad. He went into the hospital this morning, seemingly having had a stroke.

His father is at the house while Moyra is at the hospital. I will keep you informed as soon as I am told anything.

Moyra asked me to let you know.

Kristin

Alan had a biopsy that night and, with his sister Trish there to support me, the doctor told us that he was certain it was the worst of the worst, a highly aggressive brain cancer called glioblastoma multiforme. The glimmer of hope that this was just an infection was extinguished as we learned that it was cancer, and Alan had, statistically, about nine months to live.

Calls to family and friends followed. Family members, particularly my brother Don and his wife, Nancy, immediately took over all the things I normally did to help my widowed mother, allowing me to focus on Alan and our children. On the advice of a friend whose own husband had died from the same cancer, I began to send e-mails out to our family and friends. What initially served to give me time away from answering the phone and explaining the situation quickly turned into therapy for me. My virtual support group grew to include 80 friends and family members, whose support proved to be invaluable. The people you will meet within these pages are real people, not composites, and many are mentioned by name. Alan's doctors and other professionals are referred to by initial to respect confidentiality.

Friday, August 28, 1998

Hello, everyone. I'm sure you'll forgive me for telling everyone at once, but it is easier this way.

Alan has just been diagnosed with a large brain tumour. At the moment we have no prognosis. It doesn't look very hopeful. He is in tremendous pain, but his sense of humour is there and he is functioning at a high level – teasing the nurses. He is having trouble knowing what day it is but has been able to integrate sine and cosine functions for me.

We'll have the detailed results of the biopsy in a few days, so we'll know more then. I'm told the surgical access to the tumour is excellent.

Moyra

The engineer in me assumed that if Alan could integrate or differentiate sine and cosine, then his mathematical processors were intact and all was well. Sadly, this would not be the case. I stopped sleeping and eating as I tried to cope with the news. It was a very observant and wonderful nurse in the neuro-observation ward who put an orange juice in my hand and said, "Call your doctor, you are going to be no use to him if you get any sicker yourself." A few days with a sedative at night made all the difference but I was still pretty shaky. With the support of my family doctor, the Chairman of my department and my Dean, time away from teaching was arranged.

We live within walking distance of the hospital and I began to walk to visit Alan. Along the way, there is a paved path through a small woods. I used the few minutes of quiet time to prepare to talk to Alan and to his doctors and nurses. On the return home, I would decompress. On one visit, I stopped at a particular tree and told it all my troubles. The tree was a marvellous listener and I felt better for the chat. Over the next two and a half years, I often stopped at that tree to unload my worries. It didn't matter that the tree wasn't listening (or perhaps it was); the act of simply expressing my fears, worries and hopes was helpful. It was a kind of prayer, I suppose. Alan, who sometimes joked that he might well have been a Druid if times were different, actually expressed some concern for the well-being of the tree.

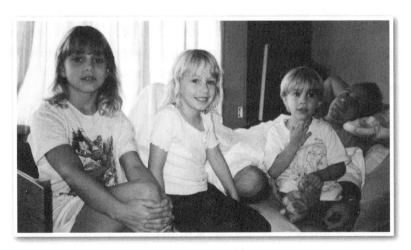

SARAH, CAROLYN, ANDREW AND ALAN IN HIS BED IN NEURO-OBSERVATION.

Saturday, August 29, 1998

First, thank you all for your calls and concern and help. We are coping as best we can. Alan is as mad as heck about this and I'm told that this is a good sign. It was one hell of a way to start the first day of our 21st year together.

The bad news is it's malignant and has probably been growing for about six months. I suppose there may have been clues about it, but they were small. Alan was sweating a bit more and was a bit grouchier than usual. The pain is much better now that the steroids he has been taking have reduced the swelling. He has no paralysis at this point but has a very weak left arm. This may improve.

Surgery is planned for Tuesday, followed by recovery plus radiation for six to eight weeks. We won't know the grade of the cancer until Tuesday or Wednesday. I am trying to be positive, but the various doctors are not saying anything at this point.

I have been given medication so that I am able to sleep and be at peace for a few hours a day. Several of you suggested this and I took your advice. Until yesterday, I couldn't sleep or eat and was too mad to relax. This really is horribly stressful, but others have done and are doing it and I will, too.

I recall waking up on Thursday morning saying, "I really don't want to go to work today." I got my wish, although I would prefer to teach ten courses per term than go through this. Your support has been a big help and I will try to keep you up to date. Fortunately, school starts soon, which should help with the kids' routines.

Alan says hi and thanks, and, for a guy who doesn't believe in God, he says your prayers are most welcome.

Moyra

Sunday, August 30, 1998

Alan wants to give you a message and he keeps asking me whether I have done it yet, so here goes. I have removed the more colourful words.

"Go home, hug your children, love your wife and spend more time with the things you love most dearly, because you or they might not be there some time."

He says that the greatest gifts of being home to work are that he has walked Sarah to school most mornings for the last two years; that he has been able to care for his sick children and see them one-on-one during those times; that he has, this summer at least, spent weekend time with them at our lake that they will remember; and that, apart from travel, we have had a family dinner (however chaotic) every night.

He is scared (I am, too) and wants you, I think, to realize that you could be in his shoes.

Moyra

Since summer camps were over and school had not yet started, I relied heavily on family and babysitters for child care in these early days. Sarah found this uncertainty very stressful but was comforted when I promised to try to come home for dinner, even if I had to go out again almost immediately. Andrew and Carolyn were less upset about the uncertainty, perhaps because their former caregiver helped more than once, taking time from her own evenings and weekends, and of course, their wonderful big sister was there, too. Alan's sister Cathy, who has four children of her own, took our three on more than one occasion. Later in Alan's illness, she would run what my kids called Camp Cathy. I would drop them off at her house for a day of total, but from a child's perspective wonderful, noise and chaos.

Tuesday, September 1, 1998

Al had surgery (a craniotomy) today. It took four hours. It was longer than expected because the tumour was bigger than the CT scan showed. It amazes me that, apart from a few bad headaches wrongly attributed to recovery from the tonsillectomy for snoring, there were so few symptoms. Now I would love to have my snoring, grouchy husband back and have no sleep again. The tumour the surgeons removed was 4.5 cm in diameter. The doctors are pleased with the surgery. Radiation five days on, two days off follows, once Alan is mobile.

There has been a lot of damage on Alan's left side, but no real paralysis. When he woke up, I asked him how he felt and he said, "I'm not going yet. I have a few nasty letters to write." He is referring to a joint paper that was just criticized, as he explained, in the usual "stupid, uninformed manner of reviewers selected from the beer halls and gutters."

We don't have the pathology even now, so the prognosis is uncertain – pretty dreadful regardless, but uncertain.

I asked the doctors when I would stop shaking (physical reaction to stress). They said, "Not for a long while."

On the upside, Alan is fighting mad. He plans to present our keynote speech in Austria next October. It would be wonderful if he could do that. He has a goal, at least.

The kids are stressed as total strangers, relatives and friends help in their care. I am trying, as instructed by those who know, to keep their lives intact as best I can. Andrew and Carolyn start back to Montessori school next week. That should even up their lives.

It is amazing how full professor, grant size, number of graduate students, number of papers, course load and all that has become so unimportant, so suddenly.

Finally, some of you may not wish to receive these e-mails. I understand that completely.

Moyra

More than once, in these early days of Alan's illness, an acquaintance, friend or colleague said something along the lines of "When one door closes, another opens."

I could certainly relate to the door closing. It felt like that door was slamming in my face and I was powerless to stop it. However, when I went home after Alan's surgery, I learned that Swiss Air flight 111 had crashed off Peggy's Cove in Nova Scotia. I realized that, unlike the families of those travelling on that plane, I had been given the blessing of time: time to prepare and time to say goodbye. The door was not actually slamming.

Of course, we were blessed with much more than time. We were blessed with two loving and extended families. We were blessed with many friends. We were blessed with my career and the benefits that came with it. We were blessed that Alan's business had turned a corner and came with benefits of its own. We were blessed to be living in Canada. Without these blessings, it would have been a very different story.

Thursday, September 3, 1998 – to office colleagues

Your fruit basket arrived yesterday and was a big hit. Andrew ate an apple the size of a grapefruit and Sarah ate lots of grapes. A visiting four-year-old cousin ate two bananas. We're all very grateful for your concern and thoughtfulness. This is a very scary time for us. Alan is very upbeat and feeling strong for now.

We still do not know the nature of the beast we are fighting. All we know is that it's bad.

Moyra

Sunday, September 6, 1998

The quiet of evening is finally here and I have taken the little blue pill that releases me from this situation for a few hours. Alan remembers a little blue pill that I once had for a severe ear infection. It made me very affectionate and he has looked for it ever since. It's possible this little pill does the same but I can't test it. One side effect of taking it to make the nights less of a trial is morning sickness! It is just a side effect but an unsettling one.

Alan is feeling very well. He had a setback yesterday in the form of a high fever, but the doctors treated it with some top-grade intravenous antibiotics and he is improving hourly. The swelling that some of you saw is sinking down his face. He remarked that he has always had a swelled head, but this time it is for real. The body absorbs the fluids slowly and gravity pulls it down so he has gone from having a puffy forehead, to puffy eyes, to one puffy cheek. The stainless steel surgical staples in his head are wild, and I'm told piano wire is holding his skull together. I'm a bit worried about these medical types sticking dissimilar metals in a saline environment so close together. The staples come out in a few days but the piano wire is there for good. I'm told it might someday trigger airport metal detectors. I hope he eventually has this problem to deal with.

He is not bald but has a bit of a strange Mohawk-style cut, with the staples making him look very punk. The droopy hospital pants add to the look. He would fit in well at the best high schools in Ottawa. I was allowed to take him outside for a walk today and we enjoyed a few hours sitting in the shade watching hospital traffic. He said that even the recently sprayed insecticide smelled good.

So many of you have called and sent cards. It is a tremendous support to us. We can't thank you enough. Some of your cards share similar stories, all with a happy ending. That gives us hope, especially me.

For those of you who have sent frozen or fresh food, thank you! However, our freezer is now absolutely full and my neighbour has the overflow and can't take any more, so please pass the word that it will be a few weeks before we'll need any more. It is so wonderful to be able to just grab a dinner and stuff it in the oven or microwave and not have to think. The kids are my focus, along with Alan, and once school starts I think the pressure will be a bit easier, since I will be able to spend more time sorting things out.

Many of you have asked for the prognosis. We don't have it yet and I'm not in a hurry. It's bad, of course, with this kind of cancer. We are hoping to be one of the ones that beat it. When I know, I'll pass it along if I have the courage. In any case, the treatment is the same. Bombard the thing with radiation and then try again if we have to. Alan is visualizing the destruction of these bad cells. He has come a long way in one week. Last Thursday he couldn't walk and was seeing double in one eye and couldn't squeeze a ball in his left hand. Tonight he walked with a walker to the waiting room and picked up each of the little guys to kiss them goodnight.

Moyra

It was important for Sarah to have her own time with me, after her siblings were in bed. It was a time of closeness for both of us and became a routine that lasted for several years. Sarah was struggling with her own uncertainties so I taught her the Lord's Prayer in the hope that it might offer her some comfort. We started saying it together every night at bedtime.

I had always prayed. I started as child, as most of us do, when my mother taught me the words "God bless Mummy and Daddy, uncles and aunts, cousins, brothers and sisters, and help me to be a good little girl. Amen." I also learned early on that praying did not produce answers in any normal, earthly sense, but that it did offer a time of quiet and a time to express, in some way, all the things that we cannot easily put into words. Often, it is a time when you learn what it is that you need or want simply by the act of expressing it, and so I turned naturally to prayer and hoped for the same comfort for Sarah.

While Sarah learned the traditional version of the Lord's Prayer, I preferred the Maori Version, from New Zealand, especially the first few lines, which seemed to be closer to my needs at the time.

Eternal spirit,
Earth-maker, Pain-bearer, Life-giver,
Source of all that is and all that shall be,
Father and Mother of us all,
Loving God, in whom is heaven:
The hallowing of your name echo through the universe.
The way of your justice be followed by the people of the world.
Your heavenly will be done by all created beings.
Your commonwealth of peace and freedom, sustain our hope
and come on earth.
With the bread we need for today, feed us.
In the hurts we absorb from one another, forgive us.
In times of temptation and test, strengthen us.
From trials too great to endure, spare us.
From the grip that is all evil, free us.
For you reign in the glory of the power that is love, now and forever.

When I told Alan that Sarah had learned the Lord's Prayer, he reminded me of the Atheist's Prayer, which he found in R. Zelazny's 1969 book, *Creatures of Light and Darkness* (Avon Books). It was a favourite of his.

In so far as I may be heard by anything,
which may or may not care what I say,
I ask, if it matters, that I be forgiven for anything I may have done or failed
to do which requires forgiveness.
Conversely, if not forgiveness, but something else be required to ensure
any possible benefit, for which I may be eligible
after the destruction of my body,
I ask this, that whatever it may be, it be granted,
or withheld as the case may be,
in such a manner as to insure my receiving said benefit.
I ask this through the capacity of my elected intermediary,
between myself and that which may not be myself,
but which may have an interest in the matter, of my receiving,
as much as it is possible for me to receive,
of this thing, and which may be in some way influenced by this ceremony.

Monday, September 7, 1998 – to a friend

Alan is feeling very upbeat. I am still scared shitless but am supporting Alan in every way I can. Today he got pissed off with the IV antibiotic pole and *carried* it into the bathroom rather than rolling it. He vows to go back and fix everything mechanical in the place some day. The wheelchairs have bits loose; the wheels on the IV poles don't rotate together.

I'll stay in touch.

Moyra

The final detailed pathology became available shortly before Alan was discharged. He indeed had glioblastoma multiforme (GBM): an aggressive form of primary brain tumour. The medical types use the abbreviation GBM. Alan came to refer to it as the Great Big Mother %$#*!.

Specimens 2 and 3. Diagnostic features are best seen in specimen #3. Areas which are markedly pleomorphic are present as well as areas with easily identifiable mitotic figures. Extensive zones of hemorrhage and necrosis are present. Again vascular proliferation is identifiable. The features are consistent with those of a glioblastoma multiforme.

I realized immediately that I was going to need to learn a new medical vocabulary. Some words, such as *hemorrhage* (excessive or uncontrolled bleeding), I already knew. Others were new to me. *Mitosis* refers to cell division; the term *high mitotic figures* became one I learned to watch for, since it indicates the rapid cell division seen with aggressive cancer. *Pleomorphic* means the tumour has various types of cells. *Vascular proliferation* refers to the presence of a significant blood supply to the tumour. *Necrosis* refers to tissue death.

Alan was released from the hospital into Home Care. The release note also indicated that he was in palliative care. I found that word very harsh and hard to stomach. Alan pretty much ignored it. Home Care covered the cost of drugs as if he were in hospital. At this point he was taking Dilantin for seizure control and Decadron for the relief of intracranial pressure.

Wednesday, September 9, 1998

I have brought Alan home to our children. It feels almost normal. Alan is doing so very well in his attitude and recovery. He looks like he should go downtown and wash car windows with a squeegee! Some of those punkers would kill for staples like Alan's.

The surgery, as you know, went very well. I made decisions for him that I would never wish to make again, such as do we take out tumour if it means he risks losing the use of his arm? (Yes!!!) In the end, he has lost little or no function. He is weak but able to walk with a cane.

Radiation follows once the incision is healed. The treatment will take about six weeks, with five days on and two days off each week. We will then see about special experimental treatment programs.

The surgeon told me Alan has a grade 5 glioblastoma multiforme. As these cancers are up to grade 4, you can guess this means it is very advanced. The current median survival time is nine months with radiation, with only a few percent surviving to the five-year mark. (As a student, Alan was always near the top of the class, so I expect great things. Also, we are told his very good recovery from the surgery is a good sign.)

Moyra

I've often wondered if, in my stressed state, I misheard Alan's surgeon or if the surgeon said grade 5 on purpose, to illustrate the severity of the illness. Perhaps it was a simple oversight, said in the stress of the moment when a doctor has to give a family this sort of bad news. I cannot imagine how hard it must be to be in that position. In any case, it was an eye-opener.

Thursday, September 10, 1998 – Alan to friends

You may by now have learned from Moyra's e-mail the grim news from the pathologist. Personally, I have never settled for being anything less than the top few percent so the statistics don't touch me at all. Some people really are too stupid to frighten. The good news is that suddenly the big bad cholesterol demon is dead, dead. I only have to worry about his bastard son, Waistline. So bring on the deep fried lard chunks. I tell people all I've lost is a couple of hundred grams of bad memories and personality flaws, two things I can easily spare. The literature urges visualizing the recovery process. I have been giving names and faces to cancer cells before tossing them down a black hole. Nothing gets out of that. If there are any special people, things or rival software packages you want to add, consider it done. They can't tell me what caused the tumour so I'm blaming it on cheap whisky and impure thoughts. Can't help the impure thoughts, so I have to buy a better grade of whisky. Life is rough. I tell all my friends to think of this as a warning. Decide what you want from your life. Spend more time with your family. No job is that important.

Alan

As part of our new family security arrangements, I purchased a cell phone that was coupled to our new home phone. Over the next few years, the cell phone was a key factor in our survival as a family. Communication was critical and it was important that the children and Alan and his doctors could reach me easily. Of course, in the first few days the new phone system didn't work and the problem was attributed to software. As our respective research work involved software development, this was quite amusing. One of the ongoing jokes that only those who knew us well understood was that one or the other of us was always finding a bug in the software on which we jointly worked.

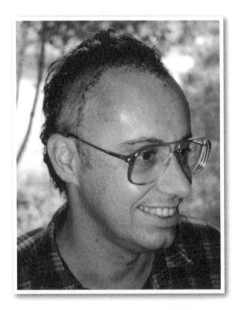

ALAN, HAPPY TO BE HOME, WITH 20 SURGICAL STAPLES
FROM HIS RIGHT EAR TO THE CENTRE OF HIS FOREHEAD.

During this time, both Alan and I were anxious to continue working on our respective and interlinked research projects – principally the development of software to predict thermal-mechanical behaviour in manufacturing processes such as welding. My goal, while I was off work and my colleagues covered my teaching load, was to complete my research grant application that was due by the end of October, fulfill my duties as a member of the university's Senate and finish a co-authored conference paper. Alan wanted to complete a number of contracts that were essential to the family finances and finish reviewing a journal paper. It turned out that he had a great deal of difficulty and required my assistance to do both these things. He had never needed me quite this way before, and it was difficult for him to come to terms with it. I did manage to complete my grant application, but we had to withdraw the joint paper. We had never withdrawn a paper before and it was surprisingly hard to do. At this point in my life, I really enjoyed the research I was doing and couldn't imagine a time that I might feel otherwise. But as Alan's illness progressed and my life changed, I began to feel that, for me, there might be something bigger than research grants and writing papers.

Monday, September 14, 1998

First, if you call the home number, don't be concerned if you get a weird message. We are setting up cell/voice mail on the regular phone line for safety reasons and there is some sort of trouble with it. They think it might be software!

You are, I know, interested in Alan's health. He is doing so marvellously well. We had, for the first time, good news of a sort on Friday. The oncologist tells us that the nine-month survival figure is for people in their 60s and 70s, so we have age on our side. Also, the speed with which Alan has recovered to this point likely means the tumour has not yet spread to other parts of his brain. (The problem with this type: it reoccurs.) We may be candidates for a special kind of high-powered, highly focused radiation after the first six weeks or so of regular radiation therapy. This should buy time for us at the very least. Again, all these therapies have risks.

Alan is miffed that he can only have a single glass of wine with dinner (or a beer). We attended his parents' 50th anniversary party yesterday. Alan had his staples out on Friday as well, so he looked more human and less like a squeegee kid. Unfortunately for Alan, it was an open bar and he couldn't partake! (Alcohol interferes with the anti-seizure meds.)

In any case, it was a day off from the nightmare for us and we all needed it so much.

He is still the same person he was, but clearly there are personality changes. Still, the math-engineering processors are completely intact (and driving me nuts, in the nicest way) but the processors that put socks in the laundry basket, clean up coffee mugs, and wipe the whiskers out of the sink seem to have been damaged (and they were never that great). However, in the scheme of things, I can live with this very easily.

If anyone tells you that health care is going to the dogs, don't believe them. We have been treated so very well and everything has moved so fast. When you are 42, have three kids and a life to live, it seems they move heaven and earth to get you the care you need. Every single nurse, doctor and staff member (physiotherapy, occupational therapy) has been wonderful.

Radiation starts next week. This week we rest up a bit and maybe try to recover from the shock. I have stopped losing weight, at least; this is not a weight-loss plan I would recommend. The immediate crisis is over for now and the kids have their dad at home to hug and kiss. I am so very, very tired.

We have a fight ahead of us that Alan is determined to win. I can't tell you how much all your e-mails and calls and gifts have meant to me especially (since Alan was out of it for a bit in there) and to the children. It seems to help them, too, to know so many people are concerned.

Moyra

The party celebrating Alan's parents' 50th anniversary was wonderful. As he did for all major family events, Alan wore his Cameron of Lochiel kilt. He looked almost himself, and for a few hours I could pretend that all was well. However, the evening also showed me the extent of the personality changes resulting from the surgery. I had expected he would sit with me, as he had always done in the past, to help with our children, especially the four-year-olds. Instead, he sat with his parents, which was confusing to me and to them. On the way home, he called me some rather nasty names, something he had never done before. I was deeply hurt. While instinctively I knew it was his illness talking, it was still a shock. Later, when I checked with both our family doctor and the social worker at the hospital, I learned that the changes in personality were likely to be permanent. I think that diagnosis was as hard to bear as the original diagnosis of brain cancer. My dearest friend had changed forever. It was to be the first of a series of irrevocable changes in our relationship. Still, I learned that we could find pleasure and comfort in the brief escapes from the reality of his illness and the stress of his treatment. It was a good lesson.

Thursday, September 17, 1998

Yesterday, Alan was fitted for the mask he will wear during radiation. The mask is really neat. They take a thermoplastic mesh and heat it in a frying pan. (The frying pan cost $700 but I have one just like it, lined with Teflon, from Zellers.) After heating the mesh, they pulled it down over Alan's face and neck, attached it to a rigid frame and let it harden in place. I must show that to my materials class sometime. You can imagine it as a hockey goalie mask. The radiation technicians showed me some pediatric masks painted to look like various superheroes. Alan has asked to have Attila the Hun painted on his.

He can breathe and he can mumble in the mask but his eyes are held shut. I gather it's claustrophobic in a big way, since his eyes must be shut and his chin is held in an unusual position. After that, the mask was used in the CT scan to do measurements for the radiation therapy. I was amused when we were told that the radiation physicists had to turn surfaces into volumes (and vice versa). That is the kind of math we do.

Tomorrow there will be a simulation of the radiation to check the measurements that were made yesterday.

Moyra

My favourite television shows at this time were medical dramas such as ER. I really enjoyed the scientific aspects of the medical diagnoses and treatments. However, immediately after Alan's biopsy, I discovered I simply could not bring myself to watch this type of show, since it was way too close to home. In time, of course, and especially when he was doing relatively well, I was able to enjoy this kind of show again. Eventually, a major character in ER was diagnosed with brain cancer. While it was difficult to watch, I was able to sit through the many episodes that paralleled Alan's experiences and understand the drama that was unfolding.

Monday, September 21, 1998

We have just returned from being summoned to the Cancer Centre for a check on the level of Dilantin (an anti-seizure drug) in Alan's blood. It's nice to sit down for a second.

Alan is doing really well. When I brought him home in a wheelchair, I had my teeth gritted for a rough ride. I had already rented a bath chair because I had been told he wouldn't be able to stand in the shower. He never used it! Within a few days, his left side had gotten much stronger and he was using only a cane. Late last week, he started walking Sarah to school.

He is grouchier than he used to be and finds the noise levels of two four-year-olds and a nine-year-old excessive at times. Three children all talking about something at the same time is a challenge for any of us. The tumour was located in his personality area, so these changes are, I'm told, normal.

In addition, there is some short-term memory loss, to which we need to adapt. Examples of this: forgetting to check before you cross the road *[That's what killed Pierre Curie, so I'm in good company. – Alan]*, leaving doors unlocked, and forgetting to put on a seatbelt. I think it can be handled with notes, although I gather it will get worse during radiation. On the other hand, Alan's math processors are functioning at a very high level. For those of you who understand these things, we had a long discussion the other day about perturbing a D-matrix using Bathe's constitutive model for better performance of the shell elements I am still struggling with.

Alan needs lots of naps and, unlike the rest of us, he can take them! *The Brain Tumour Patient Resource Handbook* (my newest bedtime reading and generally the scariest book I've ever had the pleasure of reading) indicates that sleep patterns are really messed up after surgery and during radiation. (This handbook is given to all brain tumour patients by the Brain Tumour Foundation of Canada.) So, he usually gets up in the night for a few hours and then returns to bed just as the rest of us are getting up. Again, I can live with this, I hope for 40 more years or so.

He is not able to drive for a full year, according to the law. This is true for anyone who has a seizure *[This means that the roads are safer than ever before. – Alan]*. We'll have to get used to that as well.

Alan has a scar that starts over his right ear, goes up to the centre of the top of his head and down to the middle of the top of his forehead. This flap was lifted and the bone underneath was pulled out and then the tumour, 4.5 cm in diameter, was dug out. The piece of bone was put back and is now held there with a titanium alloy. (As a materials person, I wanted to know exactly what alloy it is. I asked, but the medical types had no idea!) Then, the skin flap was stapled shut with stainless steel staples. Those were removed last week.

We have been told by the oncologist that the "resection was excellent" and the latest CT scan "looks good" with only some "granulated tissue" present. Translation: this is tissue reacting to being invaded by a knife. I used the term *brain scabs* and was told that was absolutely correct.

I have gained back half of the ten pounds I lost and noticed today that I once again have fingernails. Alan is also regaining weight. He found that the hospital food lost its appeal after a few days, let alone a few weeks. He loves the diet recommended by the tumour book. For years now I have been cutting back on fat in our diet. The tumour book, meanwhile, says things such as, "make every calorie count; use cream cheese rather than butter; mix butter in your soup; add mayonnaise to your sandwiches; eat lots of peanut butter."

Unfortunately, radiation has been delayed a week. It appears that there are some challenges associated with Alan's particular radiation dosimetry (the measurement of the absorbed dose from the exposure to radiation). However, the medical staff are doing their best. It worries us that the little blighters are in there multiplying. On the other hand, Alan is getting physically stronger each day, and starting radiation in a position of strength will be good. It has been decided that he will have five weeks (five days on, two days off) of wide coverage of the former tumour area, followed by two weeks (five days on, two days off) of focused beam radiation on the tumour bed. I hope we can then get additional treatment, perhaps a specialized radiation called stereotactic radiation, a touch of chemo or a trial of some type to improve the outcome. Every day, as things seem to be sort of normal, one or the other of us comes up against the awful statistics and has to struggle to shove those bad thoughts away. Alan does this better than I do. I'm told this is a difference in the way girls and boys are socialized. Guys externalize, as in, "That professor doesn't know what he is talking about, the exam was clearly unfair!" Women, on the other hand, internalize, saying, "Oh dear, I've let the Professor down. I should have done much better on that exam. After all, the professor taught us so well."

So, this will be a week of sort of peace, when we have only a few doctors' appointments, and we can take a deep breath and try to recover from the turmoil. Next week, we start radiation and all it brings. But we are glad to be in a position to have it. We are waiting to see how much hair Alan will lose and whether it will grow back. Alan has never been one for stylish hair.

Moyra

Wednesday, September 30, 1998

We have had a frustrating week. Alan was scheduled to begin radiation on Monday (one week later than originally scheduled) and then it was moved to Wednesday and now to Friday. We are promised that that is the last delay. The equipment at the Civic Hospital apparently couldn't handle his dosimetry and the beam pattern, and the physicist and other science types work out of the General Hospital, so it's back there for good on Friday. For now he is going to have 25 sessions of broad beam followed by eight sessions focused on the tumour bed.

If you are wondering why the delay is so critical, it's because the survival time without radiation is three to six months. A delay of two weeks is significant in terms of lifespan. On the other hand, if he is well enough to delay it, I suppose that is a good sign. He was at risk for seizures for a while. His Dilantin levels were way too low, so the doctors kept increasing the dose. Dilantin has some odd side effects, and the increase in dose affects co-ordination, among other things.

Alan continues to improve daily, and his hair is growing back from the surgery – it's nice and silvery at the temples. It will disappear again with the radiation, though. His short-term memory is improving; he now shuts doors and drawers that he opens (as least as well as he did before all this) and Sarah doesn't have to remind him quite so often to check both ways before he crosses the road. He now has an excuse for all those husband things we wives get used to but grumble about (toilet seats being left up, dark socks hanging off the edge of the bed – you know).

As I mentioned previously, his engineering processors are just fine, and we still have nightly discussions about various projects on the go and whether we should have cancelled the paper for Cancun in January. (I did, since there was no way to make the deadline.)

We have learned some other interesting things through this experience. A friend dropped off some nettle tea for me. It is supposed to be good for upset stomach (I had a lot of that for a while) and it actually worked – although it tastes a bit like drinking, well, nettles.

Another friend recommended Greens+ for energy and improved brain function. Now, as an engineer, I was pretty skeptical about this mixture of ginseng, gingko, various sprouts and royal jelly. The label says one serving is the equivalent of six cups of fresh greens! Still, we'll give it a try.

So, radiation starts Friday at 1:00 p.m. and lasts for nearly seven weeks. We are told to expect that Alan will be very tired by the third week. I'll send out another update late next week if there is anything to tell.

Moyra

It is often said that when someone in the family has cancer, the entire family has cancer. It was absolutely true for us. Simply dealing with the invasion of the constant testing distorted and affected our normal day-to-day activities. The entire family, but especially the immediate family, suddenly had to jump through all kinds of emotional hoops. It explains why I often used the word *we* when talking about Alan's illness. Clearly, Alan was sick but we all had to live with it and through it. When he had a seizure, we watched, helped with medication and waited for the effects to end. When he had surgery, radiation and later chemotherapy, the side effects affected all of us. So, while Alan had glioblastoma multiforme, we all had cancer.

Within a few days of Alan's diagnosis, I had reached out to two women, one a relative and one who immediately became a friend. Both had been all the way through this process with a loved one. Each shared her soul with me. Their stories were honest and compelling, helpful and understanding. It was the beginning of my research into understanding Alan's diagnosis and what it would mean to our family.

I had started documenting Alan's illness in the emergency room, in a small notebook I kept in my purse. As he began treatment I moved to a daily planner that I carried with me. It grew to three volumes. In those books, I recorded all his dosages, the results from his blood tests, his appointments, his doctors' names and phone numbers. I was doing it as a matter of course, but the Cancer Centre also recommends using it.

A few weeks later and feeling ready, I began to draw on my scientific training. The appropriate next step in the process was to review the available literature. I began to read. I read scientific articles in electronic and print journals. I searched the Internet. I read survivor stories and their frequently unhappy follow-ups. I read books with subjects such as living with cancer, death and dying, and the journey to death. I have since given most of them away to others but I kept two: *When Bad Things Happen to Good People* by Harold Kushner (Avon Books) helped me with the diagnosis, and *Caregiving: The Spiritual Journey of Love, Loss and Renewal* by Beth McLeod (Wiley) showed me there was a way forward.

As I learned about Alan's disease and the journey upon which we had embarked, I realized that he had decided not to be part of this particular research enterprise. The man who could sometimes be found reading scientific journals for pleasure, although he preferred history and science fiction, simply abdicated, almost overnight, the entire responsibility to me. We had collaborated as researchers for years, so I was initially perplexed by his apparent lack of interest. Perhaps not being the immediate victim of the disease, I was just a little better equipped to handle the challenges of reading about it. It helped that I had some biomedical education from my master's degree and that I had been the one who had been more proactive in learning all the potential medical issues related to my pregnancy with twins. In fact, during that pregnancy, I had participated in a hospital research study on fetal development of twins. That study had involved all kinds of testing and observations of our twins from their very early stages of development.

Thursday, October 8, 1998

Radiation has finally started. We are at the end of week one of seven. On the upside, the radiation oncologist has allowed Alan to wash his (Al's, that is) hair. Originally the doctors had said seven weeks, no washing. I gather that the metal particles in the shampoo fragrances linger after washing, which is very hard on the scalp. Alan was told to use frozen cornstarch to help clean his scalp. Now, I don't know about you, but seven weeks (even with cornstarch) would be out of the question for me. But we do as we are told in these areas. In any case, Alan asked about baby shampoo, once a week on Friday nights (he is treated Monday to Friday), and permission was given.

His scalp is getting tender where the beams go through but he has not yet lost any hair. We are told to expect three circular bald spots by the fourth week. Since Alan's hair has just grown back after being shaved for surgery (on one side), it will be quite a sight when there are three spots missing. The beams come in more or less from the top, the side and a funny angle at the back.

The major side effect of the radiation seems to be fatigue. He is sleeping now and usually does for about one to two hours after each treatment. Of course, since he gets up at about 5:00 every morning (a side effect of brain surgery is messed-up sleep patterns) he is tired by the afternoon anyway. He usually comes back to bed every morning for an hour just as the children are getting up for school.

We are officially discharged from the Home Care program as of today. That means no more therapists will visit our home for the time being. It also means that the province doesn't pay for all of Alan's drugs either. However, that is what our private plan is for. I must admit I really got a kick out of the last prescription pickup. It was for more than $500, and the taxpayer picked up everything but $2 per bottle. The private plan covered 80 percent of that, so it cost us about $1.60 for $500 worth of drugs. Next month, though, we will have just the 80 percent. However, being released from Home Care was a nice thing to have happen in the health sense, because it shows he is stronger. If Alan gets sicker it will be there for us again.

Emotionally we're doing well, but living under a death sentence takes some getting used to. Alan is still very motivated, referring to the cancer as a bloody nuisance. Sarah is a bit sensitive at the moment but is coping well. She has a better idea of the possible outcomes. The little guys are full of beans and pleased that Daddy looks better (hair, etc.) and can now play with them a bit more than even a week ago. With luck, Alan's strength will hold through the radiation. The noise levels can be very hard on him.

There is an element of powerlessness that comes with the diagnosis of a terminal disease. There seemed to be two ways to react to living under this kind of death sentence: we could surrender or we could fight. It meant the difference between a few good months and, maybe, if we were really lucky and Alan was a statistical outlier, a few good years. Most likely, it would be somewhere in the middle. Simply making the decision to fight or perhaps deciding not to surrender made us feel a bit better. Each choice that followed, whether it was to have more surgery or to enter an experimental trial, meant revisiting this decision. Ultimately, surrender might come to be the right choice.

> The other news, of a sort, is that it won't be until about four weeks after radiation stops that we will know whether the tumour, or what's left of it, is growing, not growing or shrinking. There is enough swelling of the brain tissue that it is hard to tell tumour from swelling, so the doctors can't give much information to the family during radiation.

Moyra

Thursday, October 15, 1998

This has not been a great week for Alan. The radiation started to really get to him last Friday, but by Sunday he joined us for Thanksgiving dinner and on Monday we went to the lake. It was a great day and we felt pretty positive out there in the warm sun.

Tuesday's radiation came back hard, but he was ready for that and had accepted that he needs lots of sleep to deal with it. We were trying to say things like, "Radiation is our friend."

Yesterday was a whole different ball game. Alan woke up with a blistering headache (we don't like those) with vomiting. At that point, he realized he had forgotten to take his meds the night before. Unfortunately, even taking them doubled up didn't get the Dilantin levels high enough, fast enough and by noon he had had another large seizure. I was better at it this time, having seen it in August, but it's not fun for anybody. He was able to walk (to the car) by 1:00 p.m. and we went back in the hospital to see what was up. His Dilantin levels were non-therapeutic and they have jacked up the dosage of it and the Decadron. (Radiation makes the brain swell; Decadron is a cortical steroid that counters the swelling.) So he is full of drugs today and feeling pretty low.

The other disturbing news we have been given is that there is some irregular tissue in the former tumour area that looks bad. It's too irregular to give a boost to (with a higher local dose of radiation). We also were given more grim statistics: there is about a 20 percent recurrence rate in the first year with this cancer, and an 80 percent recurrence rate in the second year. These odds are getting hard to take. We have to try and remember that statistics don't apply to us. Also, we have been referred to another medical oncologist to discuss chemotherapy options.

All in all, not such a great week here but Al can wash his hair tomorrow and usually feels much better after a day or two off the radiation. I had some counselling and will get more, I think. I need to learn how to deal with this situation a bit better, particularly how to balance the needs of three young children against the needs of my life partner. Better people than I have grappled with this, so I'll take all the help I can get.

I am trying to plan a family vacation for late November when the radiation is over and Alan is stronger. It has been suggested that this is a way of building memories for the children and rewarding ourselves for the hard work behind and ahead.

Moyra

Friday, October 16, 1998

A number of you were very alarmed by my last e-mail, so I thought I would send a weekend note that was a bit more upbeat. Alan has recovered pretty much from the seizure on Wednesday. He was full of energy at dinner last night and we had a good technical discussion as well as some chili. He is still quite tired but his energy levels are rising and he plans to walk to radiation today, as opposed to Wednesday when he needed a wheelchair to get down the hall.

The weekend always helps him feel better, since the radiation is off. After today, he'll have completed 10 of the 33 treatments.

Moyra

As we worked our way into the medical system, we learned that each of Alan's primary doctors was not only a gifted practitioner but was also, in some way, special on a personal level. Dr. A., his neurosurgeon, never failed to ask how the children were doing. This recognition, at the time of diagnosis and surgery, that we were a family, not a tumour, was among the best medical treatments we could have received as we entered this unfamiliar world. Dr. M., the radiation oncologist, was unfailingly kind, always gentle, and encouraged us to seek, and in fact helped to arrange, a second opinion. Dr. G-1, who became Alan's medical oncologist, always greeted us with a smile, a cheerful word and a kind of gruff but delightful enthusiasm. On one occasion, Dr. G-1 found Alan and I snuggled in Alan's hospital bed; we had been napping in the spooning position. With a curious little smile he remarked, "I think that's very healthy." When the news was not good, all three doctors were sympathetic and supportive. There were times, especially later in Alan's illness, when I alone received the news. At these moments, Alan's doctors became anchors in a stormy sea.

Thursday, October 22, 1998

It's been another week of ups and downs. Yesterday was awful. Today is great. I guess that is the way it will be for a while. So, back to last Friday.

We saw Alan's surgeon, who confirmed that the tumour is growing back already. In the seventeen days between the surgery and the radiation simulation, it grew from nothing to just slightly less than 1 cm. This was obviously not good news and threw us both for a loop. The surgeon seemed down but said, "Look, radiation is not completely useless! Come and see me again when it's over and we'll talk about the next phase." The fact that it has recurred so soon is really dreadful. We hope the radiation will still have a good shot at it over the next few weeks.

We then went down to radiation, trying to be brave but feeling rotten. It didn't help that Alan was still adjusting to the new medication levels from last Wednesday's seizure. I saw a social worker who has begun to take me into the next phases. One of the questions I asked her was, "Who gets priority in the master bed? The husband, whose right is clear, or the kids, who love to cuddle there?" Her answer was, "All of them. Go get a bigger bed or put a single next to the queen." So off I went to the store with the kids and now we have a bedroom that is full of bed.

Alan has the single, so as he flumps about it doesn't disturb me so much, and the kids share the queen for morning and evening cuddles. (Yes, Alan has full visiting rights in the big bed.) This arrangement works out when he goes to bed early, since the kids can still have their story with me in the big bed. If he sleeps through getting-up time, it's easier for the rest of us to leave him in peace.

Still feeling pretty discouraged from Friday, Alan woke up Saturday on the edge of a seizure. I tried out the emergency on-call oncologist and, bless our medical system, had a doctor on the phone in less than fifteen minutes and another prescription from the pharmacy *ten* minutes after that. It stopped the early seizure (shaking leg and arm) but the extra drug, really a sedative, knocked him flat on his back for the entire weekend.

On Sunday, Alan announced that he wasn't ever going to shave again. The effort of standing seemed to be too much. I pointed out that I prefer shaven men and we compromised. He now has a top-of-the-line electric razor and can shave lying down.

He was still pretty weak on Monday, so I rented a wheelchair. He cherishes his independence, so this was a toughie. However, now when he gets tired I push him along. Sometimes he can walk partway to radiation, sometimes not at all. Today, I think he'll make it all the way there, but may need to ride home. It's wonderful that we are close enough to walk. The oncologist reduced the extra medications (from Saturday) on Monday, but upped the Dilantin and Decadron again. Al also had a chest X-ray and other tests to see whether there was something else going on.

Tuesday was a bit better. The headaches are back in the morning (bad sign) but controllable with Tylenol with codeine (good sign). The social worker helped us both that day and recommended we get a few books about the cycle of life to read to the kids when the time was right. She also helped us develop strategies for helping us (the kids, Al and me) deal with his rather shortened temper (caused by drugs and surgery).

Wednesday seemed great to start with, but by 10:00 a.m. Alan felt another seizure in the works. I gather he has the sensation that his left leg and arm want to flop about. He fought it until we saw the doctor. He was given the same meds he had had on the previous Saturday to reduce the possibility of seizure. By evening he felt quite well and was able, for the first time in perhaps two weeks, to read a story to the kids at night. He even cleared the dinner dishes.

This morning has been very good. We both did some work on our respective projects-on-the-go. Alan is sleeping now and will until radiation. I have hooked up the baby monitor so I can listen for him while he is upstairs and I am downstairs. This is a comfort for him, but when he sneezes or coughs I go through the roof. Later today, we will get the results of his latest blood test and see what new levels of anti-seizure medication will be recommended, if any.

Tomorrow Alan has another CT scan. It will be a big day for us. The oncologist and the surgeon have a difference of opinion about next steps. The surgeon (being a cutting type) wants a mid-radiation CT scan so we can see how big this thing has become. As he said, you need at least two points to plot a curve. The radiation oncologist (being a radiation type) wants to wait until some time after radiation ends to see how things are going. I gather it can take months after radiation ends for it to have its full effect. However, since we are seeing a medical oncologist next week (chemotherapy type), it was decided that an extra CT scan now might give us a better picture of where we are.

CT scans during radiation are hard to read because the swelling of the brain gets mixed up with the tumour. Nevertheless, if the thing has doubled in size (from 1 cm to 2 cm), we will know that we can't wait much past the end of radiation to try the next thing. We don't even know what the next thing might be – possibly chemo, possibly more surgery with a biodegradable chemo wafer placed in the tumour site. (As the wafer dissolves, the chemo is released.) We do know that Alan cannot have the special stereotactic radiation because the tumour is not regular enough; it's a bit too diffuse. If it has stayed near 1 cm or has gotten smaller we will feel pretty good.

Several of you have asked whether I am taking care of myself. I am trying, of course. The major problem I have is that I am constantly in fight or flight mode. I have to concentrate on slowing down, on breathing slowly and deeply. Nevertheless, I often cannot seem to get my body to simply relax. I am trying a meditation tape, deep breathing, mantras suggested by various people, and the like. The best time of day for me is just before bed, when I am so tired that I know I will sleep for several hours. I relish those few hours of peace. By 4:00 or 5:00 a.m., I am awake again and it is very hard not to worry. I watch *Newsworld* and try not to think, but it's very difficult. Things get better again when the kids tumble into the bed and we all cuddle. I also relax a bit when I take them to school. I sometimes just sit in the car for a few minutes and shut my eyes after all the kisses and hugs are over.

Your support continues to sustain us.

Moyra

As the CT scan report below shows, by late October the tumour was already five times the size it had been in mid-September. It was a huge shock to learn that we had this kind of thing to deal with so soon and, again, there were more big words telling us the bad news. *Heterogeneous* means it is not the same all over; *vasogenic edema* means water is being retained in the tissue; *hydrocephalus* refers to water on the brain; *superior* is the top portion of the lesion while *inferior* is the lower portion.

```
THERE IS A LARGE NECROTIC HETEROGENEOUS MASS LESION IN THE RIGHT FRONTAL
LOBE MEASURING APPROXIMATELY 3.5 CM IN MAXIMUM SIZE.  THE LESION HAS
CHANGED IN APPEARANCE SINCE THE PREVIOUS EXAM.  THE NECROTIC PORTION
CENTRALLY WITHIN THE LESION HAS DECREASED IN SIZE AND THE SUPERIOR ASPECT
OF THE LESION IS SMALLER.  INFERIORLY, THE LESION EXTENDS ADJACENT TO THE
RIGHT FRONTAL HORN.  THE INFERIOR COMPONENT OF THE LESION HAS INCREASED IN
SIZE SINCE THE PREVIOUS STUDY AND THERE IS INCREASED VASOGENIC EDEMA IN THE
INFERIOR RIGHT FRONTAL LOBE.  THE VASOGENIC EDEMA ADJACENT TO THE MORE
SUPERIOR COMPONENT ON THE OTHER HAND HAS NOT SIGNIFICANTLY CHANGED.  THERE
IS EFFACEMENT OF SULCI AND THERE IS SUBTLE MASS EFFECT ON THE RIGHT FRONTAL
HORN BUT THERE IS NO MIDLINE SHIFT.  THERE IS NO HYDROCEPHALUS.
```

Thursday, October 29, 1998

In a few minutes I will take Alan for his 20th of 33 radiation treatments. Tomorrow he will have the simulation for the last eight high-dose boosts, with a radius of 1 cm around the tumour bed.

It has been a good week, all in all. Alan's headaches were getting very severe again, so his Decadron dose was increased, which has meant he is in much less pain. The brain swells during radiation and I gather the pain is rather unspeakable. Alan has been pretty good this week. We both managed to get some work done on our respective topics.

Unfortunately, there was also some bad news. It never ends. The tumour appears to be growing, even during the radiation. If this is so, then the doctors say it is a "real bugger." It is hard to say exactly what is happening because an ordinary CT scan cannot distinguish between blasted cancer cells and growing cancer cells. All you can see is ugly stuff, and Alan has more of that than we would like.

We have seen his medical oncologist about chemotherapy. He has offered two experimental options. There are no cures here, just experiments. The first uses a glial wafer. This would require more surgery after radiation to remove the residual tumour and to implant a chemo wafer. It would have a distinct local effect but not work on cancer cells spread throughout the brain. Apparently, this type of cancer tends to reoccur in the original site or, if not there, it will pop up elsewhere at some point. For this reason systemic chemo might be better. Certain systemic chemotherapies can penetrate the blood brain barrier but are very taxing on the patient, often lowering the blood count to dangerous levels. In other words, they poison you and hope you live.

The chemo would involve four to six 6-week sessions with the chemo part in the first two weeks and then four weeks of recovery and then another 6-week session.

The effects of radiation on Al's short-term memory are now obvious, but it should improve with time. He finds debugging code very strenuous because he can't remember what he has just done. I have spent some time with him helping him through some of this, so that he can get through another stage on a contract he is working on. He has decided that at the end of this stage, in a few days, he will declare himself disabled. His doctors support this decision. Having managed to finish a few things, his company now has enough cash to provide him with sick leave. This will carry us over until the disability insurance comes in – four months for long-term disability (LTD) but likely sooner for the Canada Pension Plan (CPP).

In the meantime, he hopes to do a fair amount of woodworking stuff in the workshop. He makes secret phone calls to Lee Valley Tools and they deliver interesting doodads and whatsits for him to play with. The doctors have suggested he not play with the radial arm saw or a chainsaw for some time!

On the upside, Alan is chuckling that he will actually receive CPP benefits before the plan goes bankrupt.

Moyra

Declaring his disability was a double-edged sword for Alan. He hoped it would give him time to do the things he always wanted the time to do, but it meant he had to face what was happening. Alan's intellect was his identity. His business and his publications expressed that identity. Still, as he struggled to do the work that needed to be done, he knew he was having trouble. It didn't help at all that I could do it. While he might have been physically ready to give up the continuous grind of providing for his family, he had been raised to be a provider. Giving up on that idea was pretty tough, even when there was some disability insurance to close the gap. Emotionally, it may have been tolerable simply because I had always been a major contributor to the family, especially when he was building his business. I, too, had been raised with the expectation that I should have a career just as my mother, a science and music teacher, and my father, a military engineer and author, had before me. I had learned the lessons of the Great Depression and World War II at my mother's knee. To some extent, both Alan and I had already dealt with the part of the equation in which I became the principal provider.

On the physical side, at least at this early stage, Alan was more frustrated than anything. He expected that his body would do what it was required to do, when he wanted to do it. However, having some physical limitations was also a logical outcome of his diagnosis, and logic was something that Alan understood. He adapted quickly to using a cane and was prepared to use a walker or wheelchair on a short-term basis. It was when he lost the ability to walk that he really felt a limitation on the physical side, but that was something we did not yet have to think about.

Thursday, November 5, 1998

It has been a good week from a number of perspectives. Alan has felt quite well, despite juggling the dosages of various drugs every few days. He has managed to walk to radiation a fair amount and has not used the wheelchair much.

Last Friday, a new anti-seizure drug was added to the set. It made Alan really dizzy, so on Saturday I made another call to the on-call doctors and over the phone we juggled the dosages. He has had very high Dilantin levels. You may recall that they used to be very low, and he had a seizure a few weeks ago. Now, they need to be lowered. The new drug, Tegratol, causes the dizziness. I have a lot of respect for these doctors, who take my reading of a situation described by Alan: "He says the room is spinning and it keeps on going even when he shuts his eyes." He says, "It is a bit like sailing but there is no boat. The deck heaves." One doctor even gave me his home phone number in case Alan had more complications. They are really wonderful people.

The effects of the radiation are easing a bit. Alan is not sleeping as much as he was, but still gets tuckered out easily. He was able to walk Sarah to school this morning. Sarah likes this, as it was something they have done together for the last few years.

He has lost a great chunk of hair where the main beam goes into the brain. It looks rather odd because it exposes the ugly scar where the craniotomy was done and it is all on one side. Alan never was much of a hair guy, though, so it doesn't bug him. As he says, he'll lose a lot more during chemo.

We attended our first brain tumour support group meeting, which was interesting. My heart went out the 20-year-old sitting beside me. He still has the surgery to go and is struggling with the diagnosis.

I have been given some anti-depressants to help control the vomiting. I have learned that the brain and stomach are more closely connected than I thought. The fight or flight reaction that causes me such trouble is normal in some people; I am hopeful that this treatment will stop the weight-loss cycle of up five pounds, down seven, up two, down four, and so on. My pants fit when Alan is doing well and fall down when he has a bad week. A nice side effect seems to be that I am getting more sleep. Now, when I wake up and realize what the situation is, I handle it a bit better.

We have learned, as I told you last week, that chemo is a long shot at best. On Monday we learned that the long shot brings an average life increase of *two weeks*! In children with glioblastoma multiforme, chemo works well. In older people, it is useless. For Alan's age group, the average is two weeks. The doctor figures it might be as much as four to six for Alan, but that is a guess. It seems like a lot of suffering to go through for an extra two to six weeks, but this will be Alan's call. I will support his choice. At the moment, he intends to fight with every ounce of his being, and I am cheering him on.

We have also learned of a new drug being tried in a multi-centre test. The problem is that it is a double-blind test and he might get the placebo. Hardly a comforting thought. We are also looking into gene therapy in Toronto. At this point, we don't know whether the gene trial is ongoing or whether he is eligible to join. We'll have to see. I guess if someone else might benefit from this horror, that would provide us with some comfort.

Alan will be going on disability insurance soon. I have spent the last few days filling out forms and getting signatures. It is very stressful to actually have to write these things down. Yesterday, I picked up the medical forms. The word *incurable* appears all over the place. Even though I was prepared for it, I felt just awful all over again.

Once he is on LTD he can apply for a partial disability, so if he is up to it, he could do some more work by summer. He really wants to work (self esteem, value and all that), but the physical limitations of exhaustion and the drug-induced fogginess are a constant irritation. I think it is marvellous that he has managed to do any work at all these last few months (maybe an hour or two each day, but some days none). It has been good therapy.

He is making each of the kids a special thing in the workshop. He has carved a hawk for Andrew and a seascape in wood for Carolyn and is now beginning something for Sarah.

We are still planning a holiday after the radiation. I will pick up a ticket for whatever we can find in the two-week period between the end of radiation and the next step – more surgery, chemo, trial drugs? There is a lot of unknown in our future, even a few weeks from now.

Here is a question for you. Are your powers of attorney in place? We had wills, of course, but an outdated power of attorney. We now have the correct ones for property and personal care. That was hard, but it does make it clear what to do and not to do under certain circumstances.

We are trying to track down the family history of brain tumours. Alan's paternal grandmother had a brain tumour, as did his aunt. We have managed to make contact with Al's aunt's doctor in Toronto. We hope to know her pathology in the next few weeks. I guess we are all worried about the familial nature of this thing, since Alan's siblings and cousins and all our children are at risk. It would be nice to have a handle on how much risk. Of course, when our kids are 40 who knows what progress will have been made?

Moyra

At this point in Alan's illness, we had brought our respective powers of attorney up to date and reviewed our wills. In addition, we sought the advice of a financial adviser to help us plan for the future. As much as I enjoyed (or did not enjoy, on some days) my career, it was apparent that financially I was going to need to continue working during and after Alan's illness. One of my priorities was to try to ensure my family's financial security.

Many of our friends re-evaluated their positions on life insurance when Alan was diagnosed. At that point, of course, it was too late for Alan.

He had felt immortal and agreed to basic disability and life insurance, seeing it as similar to fire insurance – it's there just in case and is never likely to be needed. At one point as he developed his business we had disagreed about the need for disability insurance. Fortunately, he agreed to keep it until the little ones were in grade school. It was a huge shock to Alan when he realized he was going to need it. He might have envisioned a time when his body might fail him, but never in his wildest dreams did he imagine his mind might fail him. It simply was not on the charts. Faced with an uncertain future, I began a series of steps to increase my own life insurance coverage.

Friday, November 6, 1998

I forgot to mention a few things that will amuse you. After five years of discussing the cost, Alan decided that he wanted a VCR in the bedroom. He got it. You can imagine what a husband wants with a VCR in the bedroom. However, last night we watched *As Good as It Gets*.

After five years of discussing the usefulness of the fuzzy toilet seat cover, it is now gone. Andrew had the lid fall when he was peeing. Alan has complained of this phenomenon for years and has finally won. Personally, I think the toilet looks a little forlorn, but Alan has convinced me that our son does not need a bear trap in the bathroom. Since there can be quite a mess when the lid falls down when a four-year-old is using the facility, I guess the guys have a victory here. The three girls are holding out on the seat-must-be-down rule, though.

Have a great weekend and thanks, as always, for your support.

Moyra

Thursday, November 12, 1998

It has been a much better week. Alan has felt quite well and walked Sarah to school most days. We are on the second-last week of radiation. He is now doing the boost level.

At our request, we have been referred to an expert in Toronto, who should be able to give us more information on likely experimental treatments, such as interluken and gene therapy. (Gene therapy is an experimental treatment in which genetically engineered viruses are used to carry genes and/or proteins into cells.)

It's a wild ride and our emotions go up and down like a roller coaster.

The holiday trip is off for the moment while we absorb all the information coming in from the specialists. We hope to have a family trip before Christmas.

Alan and I have had some difficult "what if?" talks. I guess we have to do that, but it's very hard. Sarah is still quite fragile but working away at school and doing well. We have had some tough questions from the kiddies. Andrew has asked, "Why is it better for Grandpa to be with God?" Sarah has asked, "How do you die from brain cancer?" Carolyn has asked, "Will Daddy die before I am a teenager?" Clearly, they have all got some understanding of the gravity of the situation.

Alan's drug dosages were adjusted again at mid-week. His Dilantin levels are now good, but the Tegratol, the second anti-seizure drug, is too low. He is learning to live on a heaving ship, since the Tegratol makes him dizzy. As he says, "I can go sailing in the comfort of my living room."

The VCR in the bedroom is great. In the evening, after the kids are asleep, we often watch a comedy. It helps to laugh.

We're off to radiation. We have only six treatments to go. Good thing, because Alan is losing hair at a fantastic rate.

Moyra

Thursday, November 19, 1998

Another week has gone by already. Today, we celebrate the last day of radiation. It's wonderful to finish the daily grind but, on the other hand, we leave the daily support of nurses, counsellors and social workers. However, as you will see, we have lots of appointments still to come.

Alan had another good week. He seems to be getting stronger as the radiation goes on. This is unusual. Most people get weaker. It lifts all our spirits when he is able to participate in things with the family, such as the daily attempts to dress four-year-olds in winter clothes when they think summer clothes are better. He had a little bit of twitching yesterday, but we now know how to stop twitches from turning into seizures without knocking him out with drugs for a day or two. The twitches were likely caused by the still-increasing, but not yet therapeutic, dose of Tegratol. Alan has given up trying to keep the doses straight, so it's up to me to count out the daily combination of pills. Today, it's seven pills in the morning, one at lunch, seven at dinner and one at bedtime. We now have an eight-week cycle of reducing the steroids for brain swelling and weekly blood tests for drug levels. It's crazy at times, and when one has short-term memory problems it's nearly impossible to keep track of the changes.

We had some disturbing news this week. We finally tracked down the pathology of Al's aunt's tumour. She had the same thing as Al does, except her GBM was in the left frontal lobe. So, it looks as if the tumour may be familial, but we don't know for sure. In any case, we will now register with the familial brain tumour study in Texas. They will collect DNA from as many of Alan's grandmother's direct descendants as they can. There are 60, I think. Perhaps it will at least lead to some scientific data that may help others.

Alan's mother took on the task of completing a family tree showing Alan's paternal grandmother's descendants. It was interesting to watch how various family groups handled the diagnosis of a third brain cancer in three generations. Some simply could not face the issue and continued as if nothing had happened. Others participated in the study and also contacted doctors to seek advice. Most of us in the immediate group finally got around to things we had put off, such as mammograms, Pap tests and tests for prostate health. The first DNA samples were gathered by taking swabs from the inner cheek. In 2004, many of us, including the youngest of Alan's nieces and nephews, had blood drawn and sent to Texas for the next level of the study. Alan had always felt that it was in the best interests of the family to do whatever we could for the science side of the disease. It was part of his motivation when deciding to continue treatment.

Of course, by this point in our lives, the requirement for scientific contribution was thoroughly ingrained. Research and publishing were immensely important to us. Participating in this study was something that we felt strongly about, especially since our children might someday face this potentially familial disease. I wanted them to have as much knowledge available as possible. The challenge of learning more about Alan's aunt's diagnosis from nearly 20 years earlier, and that of his grandmother, more than 60 years earlier, reminded me of the need to keep proper records. It was normal and even comforting to begin keeping the necessary material properly filed, labelled and documented. I had the calendar-style books for day-to-day entries. My literature review continued. I added to my files the e-mails we sent and received. I added personal journal entries and observations. I added the information sheets on his prescriptions. My laboratory logbook documenting all aspects of Alan's illness was born.

> The other grim information we learned was how this disease progresses and what stages it goes through. It's very stressful to listen to this sort of thing, but we felt we needed to know, and so the doctor did his best to tell us.
>
> In the next few weeks, we will be seeing more people. Tomorrow, we see the surgeon again to see if/when/how he wants/doesn't want to do another resection of the tumour. Next week, we will all head to Sunnybrook Hospital in Toronto to meet an expert on new technologies and experiments and drugs. Then we see the Ottawa chemo guy the week after that. Then Alan has another CT scan. At that point we will know if the tumour is still growing, has stabilized or what. Over Christmas, we will make some more decisions. It is important to find out about experimental treatments early on. Some of these are not available if you have started conventional chemo. Some require that you start the experiment within four weeks of finishing radiation. Some require a new resection and then more treatment. All of these factors have to be weighed and guesses made. Somewhere in there we will try to take a holiday.

My weight appears to have stabilized, thanks to massive doses of left-over Halloween candy, which stayed down, thanks to very low doses of anti-depressants. Sarah has been doing better lately. Andrew is fine this week but Carolyn seems to be going through a pot of trouble, which is exhibited by an inability to find anything to wear in a closet full of clothes. Oh well.

Moyra

Sunday, November 22, 1998

I'm somewhat sorry to see the end of the radiation treatments. I don't know how typical it is, but the more radiation I receive, the better I feel. Now to get irradiated I'll have to sit very close to a colour television or the rear of a computer monitor. The first is self-administered brain damage. The second is so boring it might as well be.

Alan

Alan's parents, indeed both our families, had been onside from the beginning, doing whatever they could to make things easier. One of the plans for the fall was to build a small cabin at the lake. We had purchased the property when Sarah was a toddler, and after a number of years camping there, were finally ready to build a basic cabin. Alan had planned to take time away from his contracts to build it with his brother-in-law Randy. In the end, Randy and Randy's father did it all. Of course, this had a corresponding effect on Randy's children and his wife, Alan's sister Susan. My mother and Alan's parents helped out financially to get us to the point where Alan's contracts were completed or at a milestone at which we could withdraw from them, and Alan could move to disability insurance. This meant we were able to leave our registered savings plans intact.

Alan's parents came with us to the appointment with Dr. P. in Toronto. I had been taken aside by a social worker at the Cancer Centre, who told me it was essential to build good memories for the children. In keeping with the idea of making family memories, we all went to Toronto by train, including the children. We even toured around a bit. In the hotel, we stayed in adjoining rooms so that Al's parents could babysit during the time Alan and I were at the hospital. The kids seemed to think it was a great adventure. There were times when it felt just like a nice family trip. On the train coming back, Alan didn't sit with us, but instead sat with an old friend who happened to be on the train. While they exchanged news, I took care of the children. It was a bit of a zoo and I could have used his help. However, his frustration level was such that things were often better if he did not spend a lot of time in close contact with his exuberant and lively children.

Friday, November 27, 1998

The doctor in Toronto gave us three ideas.

First, wait and see. When the tumour starts growing again, make a decision then about chemotherapy. Since standard chemo is usually useless, this is a last-ditch kind of thing. Familial tumours apparently respond to chemo better than regular tumours since they have a genetic mutation that means they don't repair DNA strands as well, but we didn't know if Alan's was familial. Also, at this point, do a new resection, fast freeze the tissues and send them off to various labs to see which chemo drugs, reo and retro viruses might be useful. Alan's case has been added to the southern Ontario grand rounds (a meeting of cancer types). The Canadians tend to be less aggressive than some U.S. centres (or so we are told), but aggressive surgery (we are told) can reduce the tumour more (but is referred to using a less gentle term: a lobectomy; sounds jolly, doesn't it?). We also learned that the gamma knife so popular in the U.S. is just a kind of stereotactic radiation treatment. Alan is not a candidate for stereotactic radiation because the residual tumour is too irregular to treat, since this treatment would damage eloquent (another nice term) portions of the brain.

Second, Tamoxifen used in low doses to treat breast cancer, can, when used in larger doses, slow or prevent growth in brain tumours (not cure or reduce, just slow or stop growth). Side effects are more or less benign, apart from blood clots in the leg (sounds nice), but certainly less than those associated with the standard chemotherapy, if you can stand taking 30 or so tablets each day.

Third, switch from Tegratol and Dilantin as anti-seizure drugs (they are very similar drugs and both aggravate the temper problem) to Epival, another anti-seizure drug also used in psychiatry to reduce rage. As many of you know, Al has always had a short temper, but it's really short now, especially with the children. And, kids being kids – "Hi, Daddy, Daddy, Daddy, Daddy! Did you know, Daddy? Daddy! Daddy! Daddy!" Jump, jump, hop, hop, skip, twist, turn, spill, crash, tears. "Daddy, Daddy, Daddy, I spilled, Daddy, Daddy, Daddy" (get the picture?) – it's hard on the kids and makes life tenser than it needs to be.

To complete the week, I got a callback on a mammogram (so, how may of you 40ish ladies have had yours yet?). One in ten women gets a callback. I figured it was just a technical problem. We less-than-bountiful ladies present a real challenge to the technicians who get their hands squished and pinched as they attempt to load the little people into the machine that suits the rest of you. My mammograms are not clear, although I am told the problem appears to be benign. Having something there is a real scare. So I am now on a breast-watch. Alan has volunteered to do this duty whenever required.

Moyra

November 29, 1998 – Alan to a friend, on disease

Now that I'm retired, I check the e-mail twice a day. I know, though, that there are people so spooked by a terminal illness that they completely withdraw all contact, either because they don't know what to say or are trying to be polite and not disturb anyone.

We have no snow yet, but it won't be long before we do. With all the appointments and such we had some trouble squeezing in a cruise but did manage. Tomorrow (today) we leave for a short, four-day cruise – Miami to Cancun and back.

My radiation treatments finished a week or more ago and I'm gradually returning to the pre-radiation sleep cycles. It's 4:00 a.m. The best thing I can do is get up, rather than lie awake trying to sleep.

As I said I'm now retired – in the sense that I don't work but merely take money from the Canada Pension Plan and the insurance company, who were foolish enough to bet that I would have a normal life span. HAH! You know how insurance works. You are betting that something bad will happen; they are betting it won't. Only bet I ever won! I cleaned up my desk and some of the directories (something I'd been putting off since retiring last month); can't say it improved my mood much. I have a great stack of inspirational books people have recommended that I read. They are less helpful than you might think. Long lists of miracle cures and touching stories of the human spirit are not my style. Me, I'll take the blood-and-guts stories.

I still feel pretty good, though there is a tendency to have headaches. I can't stand noise, which is hard on the children. My short-term memory is not great. It may come back as the radiation effects fade; it may not. In the last week or so, Carolyn has really started to enjoy playing kids' games – card games, board games, that sort of thing. Lately, she has been creaming me at a game that involves only the smallest amount of forward thinking: thinking two moves ahead to arrange a better situation than the current one to take advantage of changes made by your opponent. Beaten by a four-year-old who more or less moves at random – what can I say?

Alan

As the end of radiation approached, a number of nurses and doctors in the Cancer Centre as well as Alan's surgeon recommended we take a family vacation. While all along I knew Alan's illness was classified as incurable, the almost insistence of his medical team that we take a vacation while Alan was physically strong gave me a clear indication that we had a very rough road ahead of us. We had a much-needed rest away from the chaos and the children had a great time with their dad, especially at the beach. Alan's parents came with us. I knew already that this kind of escape, or pretending, gave us all a short respite from the realities of what we were facing. That alone was a comfort.

Sunday, December 6, 1998 – Alan, about the cruise

Thanks for all your concern and encouragement. We had a wonderful time. It was great fun. In some respects, I'm sorry to be back home.

You are right about Andrew and Carolyn. They are normal four-year-olds and full of energy and mischief. I find I can't stand the noise at times and the best thing to do is take myself out of the room and lie down for a nap. It means I get less time with them than I would like, but it's better than shouting at them to be quiet.

My mood is not all that great today.

I had another seizure while we were on the ship. Something about the vibration of the engines was the right frequency to scramble my brains. It was relatively mild, in that I was conscious throughout and I still spent most of that day and the others on the beach, but it and other signs (bad headaches, weak left arm, trouble concentrating enough to understand a simple novel, bad temper) argue that it's getting worse. Moyra is relentlessly optimistic but I think she is mostly rationalizing things. I can hardly blame her. Mostly, I regret all the things I want to do but probably won't get a chance to – that and the burden already on Moyra.

Alan

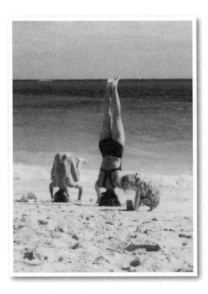

SARAH, MOYRA AND CAROLYN DO HEADSTANDS ON THE BEACH (NASSAU).

Monday, December 7, 1998

What a cruise! It's a good thing minor problems no longer cause me any stress because we had a few, but it was otherwise great. It wasn't until Sunday about 4:00 p.m. that we actually knew what time we would leave on Monday. It took two hours for the airline to sort out how to print boarding passes for a trip booked in U.S. dollars on their so-called partner airline. We really thought there were times when a pen could have been useful. You know in the old days the folks behind the counter could write a ticket manually, rather than trying to find the special (but unknown) code to deal with this partner thing.

When we arrived in Miami, a counter person screamed at us for stealing a wheelchair, which we had arranged for ahead of time. I pointed out that screaming at customers was poor PR. She screamed at me some more and then Alan shouted at her. *[Hey, I've been storing it up for years. It's only now that I have a good excuse to unload on twits in my way. – Alan]*

We nearly had nuclear war *[I had a good time; hope I ruined her day. – Alan]* but the cruise ship people pointed out we would miss the ship if this kept up so we left her red in the face but with us holding the wheelchair. Watch out for those Canadians; always stealing something.

As the ship tooted its horn, we raced (as well as one can with two cripples – that is, Al and his dad – and three kids) up the gangplank and were the last to board. Then they told us, surprise, that we were not going to Mexico. Things had changed; we were going to the Bahamas.

It was a wonderful time. They were great with the kids despite the unavailability of promised activities (broken hot tubs, playroom closed). Andrew ate mostly apples for three days, so he got the name Apple Boy (make it sound Jamaican and you have a good idea). The waiters flirted with Sarah (a bit alarming, since she is nine), and Carolyn adopted all the staff and carried out long, chatty conversations with anyone who would listen, including three nineteen-year-old guys who worked as theme animals at Disneyland and were great with kids.

We stopped at Freeport, Nassau and Great Stirrup Key. The water was cool but pleasant. I bought some floaties for the kids and they bobbed about in calm water and had wild rides (with mother cringing) in the big waves.

Alan enjoyed the beaches but sadly had a seizure the first day. He remained conscious so he now knows how awful it is to watch it happen. He recovered quickly and the ship's doctor was very helpful and adjusted his medication on the fly. Fortunately, I had a full record of his case history and he had extra meds with him. However, it is discouraging that he had another bad seizure so soon.

Alan also found the ship vibrations tended to make him feel seizurish. The vibrations were at an odd fundamental frequency for him. He usually got up and went on deck if he felt this way and so saw the launch, in the distance, of the space shuttle. He also wandered into the ship's boutique and, in his infinite wisdom, bought me a gorgeous gold and diamond necklace. This guy has always had good taste in jewels, but the three kids got a funny look as they came through customs with a full declaration each.

Apart from the seizure, I loved the trip. The kids stayed healthy, and none of us got sunburned or the trots or seasick, although there was one evening when the waves made the ship roll and Sarah and I sat in bed comfortably drugged with Gravol. I would recommend this kind of trip in a minute. Another time, I'll take advantage of the grown-up stuff such as massages and champagne. This time, I played on the beach and did headstands with Sarah and generally was silly.

Moyra

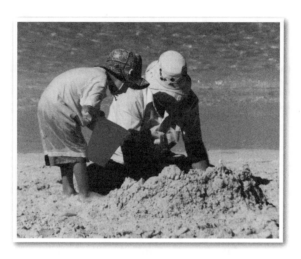

ALAN AND ANDREW SHARE THE SUN AND,
AS THEY ALWAYS DO, BUILD A SANDCASTLE (NASSAU).

Alan was referred to a neurologist to help control both his seizures and his temper. I was losing hope that we could manage Alan's anger. Dr. G-2, like Al's other doctors, was incredibly compassionate and gentle, and concerned not just for Alan but also for the family. A change in medication proved helpful.

Thursday, December 10, 1998

My family has fallen asleep and the house is peaceful and quiet again for a few hours. It has been a peculiar week, with good feelings and bad. Alan has had a slow recovery from the seizure on the ship so we checked things out with the doctors. He is quite weak on the left side again, walking with a limp and not using his left arm unless I ask him to. It is no longer natural for him to use it; he needs to be prompted. This weakness makes him very discouraged and kind of pissed off. On the upside, he is scoring very high on the cognitive scale, so the neurologist suggested we try a cocktail of eleven herbs and spices (sound familiar?). In any case, the doctor has another patient who is doing far better than expected and she is consuming this strange mixture of stuff. I was amused that a mainstream doctor would suggest this but he said, "Heck, it can't do any worse than chemo." As you may recall, standard chemo is said to extend life by two weeks.

The doctor also added another anti-seizure drug to the list, since clearly the other two are not enough. We had asked for this one some time ago, but there is some reluctance to prescribe it, since it can hurt the liver (all of them have nasty side effects). Our family doctor and the expert in Toronto had recommended it for Al because it is also known to reduce mood swings and outbursts. Al is having trouble controlling his temper with the kids and with me, too, sometimes. The kids are full of Christmas "pee and vinegar" and he has no patience right now. They are puzzled by his behaviour, especially Sarah, who is still quite fragile. The social workers have told us how to help the kids handle this, but it is hard on all of us and makes Al feel awful when it happens. He has so many good reasons for being angry, but the kids are not part of the problem. I hope this new drug will help there and control seizures. We need some help with the happies.

So, he has eight pills at breakfast, one at lunch, seven-and-a-half at dinner and three at bedtime. He is on a total of nine medications, one of which is used only when he feels a seizure coming on. Of these, one is being increased every 48 hours, one will start to be decreased in four days on a 24-hour cycle, and another is being decreased weekly, provided he can stand the pain associated with the reduction. This last controls the swelling in the brain associated with radiation and its after-effects. We reduced it too fast this week and he was in agony several times (not good for one's mood), so we backed it off and will try again in a few days. Alan has resigned himself to trusting me to do this correctly (hope I do), since he can't remember what is going on. (Alan never was good at this kind of stuff.) Having to rely on me to do this is also frustrating for him, since he has always been an independent kind of guy.

We are hoping his short-term memory will improve now that the radiation is over. So far we have seen little improvement, though. The other day, he was trying to write cheques and got really frustrated, so he asked me to do it. On the other hand, tonight we had a theoretical discussion on the merits of a modified Newton-Raphson solver versus a full Newton-

Raphson solver, including the merits of using line search. I think he won the discussion.

We are still working on documentation for his disability insurance. The insurance company sent me a letter the other day, asking for all kinds of things (I had already sent about 25 pages of documentation), including a requirement to "fill out the enclosed form and return immediately." There was no enclosed form. Several calls later, I reached a human who told me to send his file. I asked, "All of it?" She said, "Yes." The cost of getting two pages of one's record from the hospital is roughly $5. Getting a medical form filled in is about $50 (if the doctor has to sign it). Alan's file looks like one volume of an encyclopedia now – I have seen it. The cost of copying it boggles the mind. In any case, after suggesting she tell me more precisely what she needed, she allowed that perhaps five more pages would be enough.

Moyra

Monday, December 21, 1998 – Alan to a friend

I'm now awake. As often happens with brain injuries, my sleep rhythms are totally screwed up. I sleep for no more than four hours at a stretch. I get up at 4 a.m. every day. Seeing the sunrise is lovely, but this is not what I meant when I wished I woke earlier to enjoy the best part of the day. It also means I conk out in the early afternoon for a nap. Be careful what you wish for, I guess.

My radiation is over now, too, which is something else I miss. The more rads I got, the better I felt. With all the stories about long waiting lists for treatment in the Canadian medical system, the speed with which I've been hustled through says something I'd rather not think about.

Apparently surgery works on GBMs and so does radiation, but the best chemo treatment extends survival by two weeks on average. I'd like to know how they would be able to tell if it were useless. Must be tough to get below zero. The side effects apparently are severe enough that blood counts are ruined to the point that many people can't finish the course of treatments. More good news! What little reading we have done says GBMs grow fast and are highly invasive. The tumour can be in one hemisphere with tendrils growing across to the opposite side. (I guess my warranty was for only 20 years of marriage.) The location was in what the doctors say was not an eloquent part of my brain. This means that when they removed it, all I lost was some bad memories and personality flaws. Those I can spare! Many people have suspected that I was only using a very small part of my brain anyway. It has often been said that disease goes for the weakest organ. Speaking strictly for myself, I can't argue.

I still have my irritating sense of humour, much to many people's disgust. I have decided that my cancer was caused by cheap whisky and impure thoughts. I can't do much about the thoughts, but for damn sure I'm buying a better grade of whisky. Now that I have recycled all the jokes I've been wholesaling, I'll get back to serious stuff.

With the seizures, I'm not allowed to drive. I tire quickly enough that I don't walk far. The weather is turning crappy here, anyway, so I spend a lot of time at home, inside. I'm afraid that talking to me is a bit like lancing a boil. You may get more than you want and not know how to turn it off.

One thing I've noticed is that everyone I speak to has a story of some relative with exactly the same thing (cancer of the elbow or some such), who went somewhere (Las Vegas or Baghdad or whatever), took something (coffee enemas, Mocha-Java please, lots of cream and sugar) and had a miraculous recovery. It's irritating, but they mean well.

Alan

Tuesday, December 22, 1998 – Alan on faith to Bob, a U.S. colleague

I've been finding the book you sent quite thought provoking, as I hope you intended. I was a little disappointed with the quality of the arguments put forward by the atheists. To get suckered into the most basic traps shows little imagination. Proving that something didn't occur or never existed is difficult, not to say impossible, unless your standard of proof is so sloppy as to be worthless. At best, you can only say that the evidence showing its existence hasn't appeared yet. One might argue that it appears to violate some physical law, like conservation of energy, but any halfway talented magician can do that. They might argue that there is no evidence proving the existence of a god, but a supernatural being capable of creating the universe would, I would think, be able to remain hidden if it wanted. With no evidence to prove its existence and no way to prove its lack of existence, the question is now what do you believe – a matter of faith or lack of it?

Some of us are incapable of faith, just as some of us are colour blind. You tell me there really is a colour. You tell me this dog or that flower is coloured. I can't see it, and I can't prove that you don't. If enough people agree that such a colour exists, then, whether it exists or not, I am forced to admit that you live in a richer, more colourful world. This much I can prove. I can't see the red berries on our currant bush or the purple crabapples on our tree or the raspberries when they are ripe amongst the green foliage.

Alan

I don't recall that Alan or I ever said, "Why me?" through all of this. Alan did wonder why not a few others – say mass murderers – but he rarely questioned, at least aloud, the unfairness of it. He was more likely to say simply, "Shit happens." We both understood that someone has to get these things and that on a statistical level the question was, more correctly, "Why not me?"

There was a difference, though, in where we went after asking that second question, both in terms of faith and in terms of science. He and I had long ago agreed that I could believe in a higher power if I wished. In fact, I think he regarded my faith as a rather quaint, and perhaps endearing, weakness. So while I was able to seek comfort from my faith in something like the Earth-maker, Pain-bearer and Life-giver of the Maori prayer, Alan could not. Alan believed in Alan and assumed, quite simply, that he would receive medical care that was based on the very best science. I was determined to use that same science to slow the progression of his disease.

Since Alan placed his faith in himself, it was only by sheer willpower and the knowledge that those speaking meant well that he remained calm when told to "take Jesus into your heart and save your soul." Alan was aware that those with deep religious faith were not immune to cancer or to other human frailties. When the children were baptized, at my request, his comment was something along the lines of "No loving God would damn a child for the lack of a few drops of water." In terms of his soul, should he have one, he had similar thoughts. In simple terms, Alan was prepared, if necessary, to argue the merits of his case, in person, with St. Peter at the Pearly Gates.

Despite Alan's lack of faith, he did ask me several times to make sure the children received more religious education than he had. While this appears at first glance to be a paradox, it was simply that while Alan believed in Alan, he knew that the children would not have Alan, and so perhaps they should have something else to fall back on, just in case.

Tuesday, December 22, 1998

I had said there would be no further mail until January, but a number of you know that Alan had a CT scan last week and are anxious for news. We saw his medical oncologist this morning and we now have the opinion of the radiologist. I have cut out the medical terms. In short, "There is significant growth of the existing GBM."

Although I think both Alan and I thought this might be the case, it still upset us both. You always hope you are exaggerating the worry. The loss of innocence is awful. We used to always say to ourselves, "How bad can it be?" Then you find out just how bad it can be.

For the first time, I cried in front of the doctor. Even he looked miserable. What a time of year to have to give this sort of news. Alan just looked at the floor a lot, wondering, I guess, what else they were going to slam him with. There is still likely some brain edema (swelling of the tissues) from the radiation, but the growth of the tumour is the shits from many perspectives. Clearly, this thing isn't stopped much by radiation. Tonight I will try to explain to the kids the next level of their daddy's illness. I guess I'll cry some more then, too – poor little things.

Further surgery is another option, but at what cost? One could debulk (neat term, isn't it?) the tumour but the surgeons tend to be as aggressive as possible the first time out. Next time round, paralysis? We will see a surgeon again for an opinion and e-mail the guy in Toronto to say that the recurrence is already upon us. He had some ideas for other chemo treatments.

For the moment, Alan is going to start conventional brain tumour chemotherapy right after Christmas, in the first week of January. We have learned that familial tumours and those in small children *[Let's hope that includes the infantile! – Alan]* respond better than others to chemo, so it is a shot we have to take. His quality of life should be relatively good through the chemo, although he will be at risk of infection, especially from the kids (two schools and all their germs) – not to mention the nice university-level bacteria I'll pick up.

I hope I haven't ruined too many Christmases and other holidays by this note. I know some of you were waiting and hoping with us. I wish I could tell you something different. I wish … Oh, I just wish. We thank you, as always, for your support and love and concern and prayers. Remember it is not the line at the checkout, or the size of your paycheque or the jerk driving in front of you or the long commute that matter. *[But all these things* are *important! – Alan]*

Our fight is not over yet, not by a long shot. As it says somewhere in the Bible, "Whatsoever thou chooseth to do, do it with thy might." *[There are others. My favourites are from Monty Python: "Removeth thou the pin from the holy hand grenade and count to three. Thou shalt not count to two; neither shalt thou count to four." – Alan]*

Moyra

Christmas had always been a very special time for us. I had loved the holiday from early childhood with church and parties and feasting and presents. In hindsight, of course, I realize that my parents found it very stressful, but to my childhood eyes it was a time of wonder. To my delight, Alan's family had large and enthusiastic Christmas gatherings, with carols belted out during after-dinner dishwashing.

Alan and I merged our Christmas traditions easily when we married. Our families came from largely English and Scottish backgrounds, although Al's includes a Cree heritage, of which they are very proud, from the early days of the Hudson's Bay Company. All four of our parents had grown up in Winnipeg and attended the same university, although at different times. Fathers and grandfathers on both sides of the family served their country during war. Christmas, for us, meant, above all, time spent with the family. There was, of course, Christmas Day itself, with all the excitement of presents and dinner, but there were other events that continue to this day, such as family bowling night. Christmas music was a key part of the tradition and, for me, there was church and worship. By focusing on family, we avoided some of the commercialization that surrounds Christmas, and the music told the many stories of Christmas, from Christ's birth in a lowly place to peace on earth.

This Christmas, a social worker at the Cancer Centre explained, might be our last together. I should make it special and continue to build memories for the children. I had heard this message of building memories already. I suppose the idea is to bank memories for the future so they can be withdrawn as needed. When you expect to have a future, you know these memories will be built as a matter of course. There will be family vacations and other events to provide these memories. As an expert of sorts in my own discipline, I accepted the learned expertise of those in this discipline. What I hadn't expected, but was learning, was how much effort it would take to build those memories for the children. I wish the social worker had also told me how difficult it would be, both emotionally and physically.

At the candlelight Christmas Eve Service at our parish church, I enjoyed a few hours of quiet peace while Alan and the children slept at home. In that environment of families worshipping together, my prayers for my family were heartfelt.

In the end, this particular Christmas was not wondrous or boisterous, at least not for me and certainly not for Alan, who frequently had blistering headaches. Nevertheless, the children do indeed seem to have good memories of gifts and family feasting, so we must have been at least partially successful. It was a very challenging time, as Alan's next letter shows.

Tuesday, December 29, 1998 – Alan on children at Christmas

I have been finding, now that I am retired, that getting and responding to messages is the highlight of my day. I shall assume the same is true for you. The self-help books urge you to see the positive side of cancer. Apart from knowing I'll miss the Mayan end of the world in 2012 and the big asteroid impact in 2028, I find the surgery and drugs must have shaved at least 20 points off my IQ.

We had a traditional holiday here. "Andrew, stop jumping on the couch. Carolyn, don't call Sarah old Poo-poo face. Sarah, I don't care what he did, don't hit Andrew. THE NEXT PERSON TO PULL ANYONE'S HAIR WILL SPEND THE REST OF THE MORNING IN THEIR ROOM. Yes, Moyra, perhaps I should have a nap."

Alan

Many friends said to me, "God only gives you what you can handle," but, actually, it is sometimes more than one can handle alone. I found that reaching out to family and friends was critical. During these early months of Alan's illness, there were times when the temptation to stick my head under a blanket and never come out was palpable. If I could have hidden under a blanket, I would have! I understand, on some level, those who cannot cope and choose to simply pretend it is not happening, those who bail out or move out, or worse, under the load or the diagnosis, the long or short treatment, and everything that follows.

It was heart wrenching, and at times almost crippling, to watch the decline of this man who was so much of everything to me: husband, research partner, best friend, breadwinner, lover, comedian and father of our children. I cannot explain how awful it was to be asked to hold him down during a seizure and try to help him cope with the various indignities that came with the seizures, especially the really bad ones. I felt so very sorry for both of us. I could not comprehend how I was to go forward, nor where I would end up.

I knew, though, that I had made a commitment to this man and that I loved him. One afternoon shortly after he came home from the hospital, I remember being very frustrated and very angry and saying to him, "My husband has brain cancer. I'm going to be all alone. How do you think I feel?" Alan responded equally vehemently, "I'm the husband who's dying. How do you think I feel?" We just stopped and looked at each other, realizing in one awful moment the depth of the other's hurt and confusion. In the past, we had faced things together: his depression, my difficulties becoming and staying pregnant, and all the other turmoil of life. Now, for the first time, neither of us could make it better for the other. I think it was that day that I really acknowledged deep down inside that I had made a vow that contained the words "for better, for worse; for richer, for poorer; in sickness and in health." I determined that somehow I would keep my vow. I was going to have to find a way to establish control when things seemed out of control. I was going to have to learn a new way of caring and a new way of loving.

It was a white-knuckle sail from day one. There were times when only that vow and my responsibility to my children kept me going. There were times that only having family and friends out there kept me going. Friends and family would show up with a bag of groceries, a bottle of wine and a hug. Friends and family would welcome me for a cup of tea when I arrived at their door to pick up my children. A neighbour seemed to know when to invite my children over for an afternoon of arts and crafts. Parents of my children's friends became friends and supporters. There were those who agreed to watch my children for a morning and ended up keeping them until late in the evening as a setback turned into a crisis. Relatives and friends drove my children to and from their activities without complaint. This network of friends and family sustained me. I don't think they will ever truly understand the depth of that support. Every offer, every prayer, every letter, every e-mail, every hug, every drive for one of the children, every cup of tea – and there were many – made it all just a little bit more bearable. As I faced the reality that I could not do it alone, I learned to ask for help when I needed it, and I tried to accept help when it was offered.

Each crisis was handled in turn, driven by endorphins and adrenalin, and other interesting bodily functions. In many respects, the day-to-day problems were harder to manage than the crises. When I felt overwhelmed, I learned to stop and just breathe, slowly, in and out, allowing myself to simply count – nothing more. I would get through the moment, then the minute. I would count my blessings: I am healthy, the children are healthy, we have a home, I have a career, I have medical benefits, there is enough money, we have friends to help us, we have family to help us. As calm, or strength, returned, I would face the next hour and then the day.

I drew strength from my experience of being a mother of newborns, especially of twins. During those first few sleep-deprived months of motherhood I dared not think about the next week or month. I would simply aim at some undefined future time and promise myself we would take each thing as it came. I remembered my father's diagnosis with Alzheimer's and my mother learning how to cope. I remembered my undergraduate and graduate school years in engineering and all the hard work and hours of studying. I reached back to my teenage years as a high school athlete, when I had learned that perseverance was required to be successful. Perhaps even more important, I remembered that while I won some races and lost many others, I had never bailed. I reached even further back to my childhood and growing up in a home that always had some ongoing major construction project, with siblings and parents coming and going with their own lives. All bundled together, these experiences allowed me to face the unknown, but virtually certain, outcome of Alan's illness.

2

January to April 1999
CHEMOTHERAPY
AND THE SECOND RESECTION

After much thought and advice, Alan chose to take the standard systemic chemotherapy, in part because it would treat the entire brain. His cognitive losses were becoming plainly evident to me, but not so much to those around us. I found myself mitigating and covering up his errors and, in some ways, protecting him and his family from the true extent of his illness. I suspect it is a natural thing to do for one's partner, but it was especially important to do it for Alan, who felt his intellect was his identity. Unfortunately, that very vulnerability seemed to make him even more determined to be the person he had always been. He became very frustrated when he could not do something he thought he ought to be able to do. My doing things for him only added insult to injury.

Emotionally, Alan was often on the edge of anger, and there were a few times that I was actually frightened by the extent of his anger. The blunt truth was that he had every right to be angry. I never found a good strategy to cope properly with his anger at me or at his situation, but I knew it was better that he express it to me than to the children. I at least had an adult understanding of his helplessness. Sometimes, one or the other of us managed to walk away before voices were raised. More frequently I just let it roll over me like a big black cloud, but even that left me all knotted up inside. It was a no-win situation. Fortunately, I knew without question that he loved me and that he loved the children. Somehow, just knowing that made it a little easier to get through.

As we moved into this next phase, my background in research proved to be useful in Alan's treatment. I increased my reading of scientific and medical material and continued to build my logbook of data, observations and experiences.

Tuesday, January 5, 1999 – Alan to a friend

I shall be starting chemotherapy very soon now. I'm told that familial tumours respond better to chemotherapy because there is already some problem with the cell-division process that caused the cancer and that makes it more vulnerable to insults. Sounds like doctors desperately grasping at straws to keep presenting some hope. (Of course we don't even know if it's truly familial.) We did overhear one doctor talking to his assistant about always being certain to give the patients some hope. Then he walked into our examination room. Credibility has been reduced somewhat ever since, but I shall try to play along. Don't want any negative placebo effects. The progression for this disease, I'm told, is more headaches, more seizures and, as the internal pressure grows even stronger, a gradual reduction in mental activity, gradually becoming more sleepy. So far, at least, I have been getting worse headaches and more seizures but increasing dosages of various medications has kept things under control. I hope that your time away from the city allowed you to resolve some of the difficulties. In many ways, problems like this are worse for the parents and siblings than for the victim. I'm told my brother is having a lot of trouble reading our regular messages. My mum is quite upset, too. Courage is something you have had to demonstrate as well.

Alan

Wednesday, January 6, 1999 – Alan, on not knowing what to say

I appreciate the difficulty in knowing what to say. Really, just knowing that there are people out there who want to know and who don't mind listening is a big help. There really is nothing much to say. Mostly it's important to keep optimistic, which is admittedly harder to do some days than others. I started chemotherapy today. No beer for fourteen weeks! This better work or I'll be back for a refund. Every day, I find new impairments. It's surprising how many ways you can get your arm caught in a sleeve. Algebra is a lot tougher, but spatial manipulations are now nearly impossible. I tried to write four cheques off the company books the other day and made mistakes on two of them twice!

Alan

Wednesday, January 6, 1999

Thank you all for your support over Christmas, particularly the funny notes you've sent to Alan. I am still having an argument with one of our friends, Jed, who claims that pulling nose hairs for a guy is more painful than labour for women.

As you know, the disease is progressing. The tumour is larger but we do not yet know how much, only that it is significant. With the new amalgamated hospital, Alan's charts move around and around and always seem to be in the wrong place. It appeared that chemo would be delayed, but when we told the oncologist we saw on Monday, he said he would make it happen. Alan asked him if he "knew someone." His reply was that "he was someone." As a result, Alan starts chemo today.

One great part of the new amalgamation of hospitals is that we can get the chemo at the General, while the doctor is at the Civic. Since the General is in our backyard, we prefer the General site. We hope the familial nature of this tumour will be on our side, even though it has not been confirmed as familial. Chemo often works better on these types of tumours. If it makes him too weak or makes his life absolutely awful, we will reassess the situation. The routine looks like this: six 6-week cycles. Each cycle consists of a hospital IV on day one, oral at-home chemo on days two to seven for the first two weeks, and then four weeks of recovery. The next CT scan is after three cycles. We have access to home nursing during this period if the nausea becomes really bad. They have a new miracle drug that is supposed to keep upchucking under control. Sometime in the next little while, we'll also see a neurosurgeon about another aggressive resection and all that that might entail. Alan is not keen on this if it means paralysis or some other major impairment.

Our moods swing from hope to despair, but that is normal. I can see the progression of the illness. At the moment, Alan has little seizures every two days or so. Fortunately, we have some medication (Ativan) that almost always stops them before they get really awful. I am amazed at how calm we have all become when this happens. Alan called up to me on the weekend and I came down quickly to meet Andrew coming up to tell me, calmly, that Daddy needed me right away. It was a pretty bad but still mild seizure. Alan was shaking on the floor, but the medication was under his tongue and it stopped the seizure progressing beyond the arm, torso and head, and he was able to talk throughout. The kids were super. They got a blanket for Daddy and sat quietly waiting for me to stop helping him. Not that there is much I can do, except hold his hand and talk in a calm voice to distract him. If he loses consciousness I just roll him on his side to prevent choking.

The new anti-seizure medication has helped his temper quite a bit. We will need to add another medication this week, because the little seizures are getting too close together and that means adding to the combination of drugs. I'll let you know how the chemo goes.

By the way, if you find these letters too hard to read, or would rather not know anything more, please feel free to tell me and I'll remove you from the list. I certainly do not want to add trouble to your lives.

Moyra

Andrew and Alan had been playing some sort of game together in the family room when this particular seizure started. It forms Andrew's single strongest memory from his dad's illness. It must have been very frightening for Andrew, at not quite five years of age, to be sent to get his mummy because although his daddy was talking he was also flopping around on the floor like a fish out of water. Since Alan had sent Andrew to get me, I knew Alan felt he needed adult help. For a while, Andrew was nervous to be on his own with Alan, just in case there was another seizure. In time, of course, seizures, mild and severe, simply became a part of our existence and the children and I became quite good at handling them and his post-ictal (after-seizure) recovery. We began to understand what might trigger seizures. Fluorescent lights, especially at night, seemed to be a trigger, so we replaced all the fluorescent lights with incandescent lights. Being overtired also seemed linked to seizures, so we tried to be sure Alan had plenty of rest. Certain motions, like those used to butter toast or move pieces on the checkerboard, also caused seizures, but were harder to eliminate from day-to-day life. The computer screen and typing could also trigger a seizure if he was typing too quickly, so he had to do that kind of thing carefully.

Thursday, January 7, 1999 – Alan, on faith, to Bob

I am still chipping away at the book you sent. It's slow, partly because of fatigue and some impairment, mostly because I feel some time pressures. There is so much I want to complete and the time available is uncertain. If you can stand a page-by-page assessment of the ideas, I'll keep reading it and writing to you.

It is quite true that our mental attitudes and expectations may well interfere with any relationship with God, which is something I had not thought of. For me, obedience has always been a problem. When I was small, one of my teachers used to read Bible stories every day. She chose the stories – always Old Testament – so we were treated to Exodus, Job and the two guys who got drunk in the church and were killed for blasphemy.

It seems now that my attitude to God has always been a lot like being swept up by a Royal Navy Press Gang and left with someone who, with the lash and noose, would control every aspect of my life, like it or not. Obedience could be enforced through threat of pain, but this is no way to acquire allegiance of affection. So it has remained, with me too stubborn to give in.

I can't really say I have felt a need for a reason for my suffering or anyone else's, especially since the Swiss Air flight crashed the same night as my surgery. These things happen. Life is uncertain, it always has been. By comparison, I've been lucky.

Alan

As the virtual support group of family and friends grew, Alan connected with a cousin on his mother's side of the family who also had a brain tumour. Even though her tumour was technically benign (atypical petroclivial meningioma that had invaded the clivus bone, which is located in the centre of the cranial floor), her surgery and treatment were similar to what Alan received for his malignant tumour. Janet and Alan exchanged e-mails throughout his illness, since they faced many of the same challenges. Janet went on to participate in a support group and is an active survivor and supporter.

Thursday, January 7, 1999 – Alan to a his cousin Janet

No, it isn't just beer that is verboten. It's alcohol, in all its disguises, and it's not for fourteen weeks, Moyra tells me; it's for 28 days (twice fourteen days). I was never good with numbers; that's why I became an engineer. Lucky for you, I've never designed reactors, aircraft or even kitchen utensils. The great thing about software R&D is that in the unlikely event that anyone reads the papers published in my name, they probably won't understand them anyway.

From the sounds of things, my disabilities are not worse than yours, so complain all you like. Misery really does love company. I may have it bad but, poor thing, you have it worse. In fact, I wish I felt this good back when I was healthy. Numb fingers would be a real bummer. Me, I'm just clumsy. It took me 40 years to learn how to tie my shoes properly. Did you know that the knot you tie is supposed to be a standard reef knot using loops of lace for the second right-over-left knot? When done properly, they don't undo nearly as often. Here, for 40 years, my laces have been coming apart because they were just tied with granny knots.

Back to the symptoms: getting up at 4:00 a.m. is one of the highlights. I've always wanted to see more of the early morning. I meant in June and July, of course, but January will have to do. If it means I sleep in the morning and afternoon, then my days haven't changed all that much. Now I'm unconscious upstairs, instead of in front of a computer. I'm surprised that there are enough brain tumour patients in South Florida to hold a conference. Must be due to the large number of Canadians infesting South Florida.

Alan

At various times throughout Alan's illness, he received Home Care and his medications were covered by the provincial health care plan, as they would be if he were in hospital. He was also eligible to receive physiotherapy and/or occupational therapy at home. From time to time, as his status changed, I would have to run interference to make sure that all worked out as it was intended. Running interference often meant having the local pharmacists onside. They were always helpful, but especially with respect to making sure I knew the changes in doses and helping to identify possible side effects and interactions. They were an essential part of Alan's support team, as the e-mail below shows.

Tuesday, January 12, 1999

Alan started chemo last week, as you know. So far, the cycle has been good (touch wood, salt over left shoulder).

I had some fun at the beginning trying to get the doctors, Home Care and the drugstore all on the same page at the same time. The doctor forgot to tell Home Care what we were getting and forgot to fill out one form covering one drug. The drugstore informed us that the province no longer covered the cost of one drug and that we couldn't get the other until the doctor filled out the form. Several faxes and phone calls later, it was all sorted out. The province does cover the drug, since the generic is not available (error at drugstore) and the miracle anti-nausea drug cost ($25 per pill, mind you) was covered after the doctor filled out the required form and faxed it over.

On Saturday (yup, the weekend), I finally got a call from the neurologist (my kids and his were the common background noise). Al's anti-seizure drugs levels were raised again, so back I went to the drugstore. Every time the owner sees me, his trip south becomes more of a reality. He is very attentive and helpful when I arrive with six or so new prescriptions to be filled. While Alan is on chemo, the province covers almost all drugs. Between times, my private plan and my bank account cover the rest.

Unfortunately, the chemo is associated with some rather severe food restrictions. Here are a few: absolutely no alcohol, no aged cheeses, no moldy cheeses (Al loves blue cheese), no broad beans (there go lima beans – yay! – and chili), no pepperoni, salami or bologna, no sausage, no pickled herring, no fermented anything, no banana or banana peel (the latter is not a favourite of mine), no meat or fish, poultry must be very fresh, no brewer's yeast (there go the de-alcoholized beers and wines), limit milk, limit berries. It goes on and on. Worse, he can't have any alcohol until two weeks after the last chemo pill goes down. So of all Alan's vices, he is left with only one … and kissing is out, too.

The culprit in these foods is tyramine. Normally, an enzyme called monoamine oxidase breaks down tyramine. However, one of the components of this particular chemotherapy inhibits the enzyme, allowing tyramine levels to rise. The unpleasant side effects run the gamut from dizziness to intracranial hemorrhage (bleeding inside the skull).

So, it's been a good week, finally. We hope his blood counts will be strong enough to continue with the IV this week. We have to really watch for germs. The nurse explained it like this: no kissing the kids or your wife or anyone else, either. The kids and I must not sneeze, cough or throw up on Alan. We disinfect doorknobs, light switches and taps often, and wash our hands before and after everything – this is hard on the boys in the family, who are not big on hand washing. Since stomach flu is in Andrew and Carolyn's class, we are waiting to see if it gets into our house.

Moyra

Tuesday, January 19, 1999 – Alan, on being competitive

Yes, it's been a real shock. Odd how it affects different people in different ways. For me, it's like it happened to someone else. Apart from feeling a lot of time pressure to complete a lot of things, I can't say it has been terribly upsetting. I tell people it's because I'm too stupid to be frightened. Others mistake this for courage. What I have is officially called glioblastoma multiforme, GBM (a.k.a. Great Big Mother #$!@%*), the worst kind of brain cancer there is. Nauseating, isn't it, how competitive some people are? Not only got to have the worst disease but treats life like it's a race and is trying to get across the finish line first. Stupid bastard! I guess its true that disease always goes for the weakest organ in your body.

The doctors are very careful, when I ask what the survival statistics are, to point out that statistics don't describe individuals. True enough but it's individuals that make the populations described by the stats. I have been doing my best to get into a population separate from the one used to collect the dismal survival stats. Since many victims are in their 60s, I am already in a different group. My general response to surgery, radiation and chemo has also been very encouraging. Immediately after surgery, I was back to normal. The more radiation they gave me, the better I felt. So far at least, there has been not a hint of nausea from the chemo. Besides, I have a keynote address to deliver in Austria next October. I worked too long and hard to miss that.

Alan

Wednesday, January 20, 1999

Well, Alan has finished the active drug part of cycle one of six cycles of chemo. It wasn't too bad, but the fatigue is getting to him now. Like all of us, but especially you guys, he hates being weak. He has two weeks of dietary restrictions to go and then two weeks when he can enjoy the occasional beer and then back on the chemo again. During this period, a VON nurse visits once a week to check on him.

Last night at about 1:00 a.m. he announced to me that he was going to beat this thing and then rolled over and went back to sleep. I didn't! His sleep patterns are quite strange. Up for two hours, asleep for two, up for five, asleep for four. I never quite know when he'll appear and disappear. He does make an effort to be with us for breakfast and dinner.

His hair is growing in slowly over the radiation area. I am pleased to see the scar a bit more hidden. Of course, he is likely to lose all his hair again as the chemo gets going. I'll send another update in about two weeks or so, as we get ready for the next cycle or if the news from any of his doctors is worth repeating. We still see these folks fairly often, although things are a little quieter now as we go through these chemo treatments, which are done largely at home.

Moyra

Monday, February 1, 1999

It's been a pretty quiet time since my last letter, with not much to report. Alan has been quite well, sleeping a lot, but cheerful for the most part. He has had only one seizure in the last ten or so days. Getting the chemo drugs out of his system seems to have helped, as has another increase in his anti-seizure drugs. During chemo he was averaging one episode every 24 hours, and that is distressing.

The last seizure took place in the bathtub. Alan always carries the miracle seizure-stopper in his pocket, but it's kind of tricky to do that in the bath. So there he was, bathing, when it started. Of course Sarah was in the room as well, using the toilet (big rush and the other toilets were simultaneously occupied, we can seat only three at a time – makes me wonder how our parents survived with one toilet and four or more kids). Despite our best efforts to keep them out of the way, in the space beside the tub were two stools to reach the sink for brushing teeth. The stage was set.

Alan said, "Uh-oh" and my training as a sprinter-hurdler came into good use. I hurdled down the hall over toys, a small warrior encampment not yet cleaned up and other household paraphernalia and into the bathroom to find Alan half in and half out of the tub, trying to get the pill into his mouth but having lost most of his hand and arm control. Sarah was unable to help (too busy on the toilet) but was struggling over to him with her pants around her knees. Although she has never given Alan the pill, she knows how and when to do it. Andrew finished up where he was and appeared to help, too. So there we were, four of us, in a small family bathroom. Thank heaven the cat and Carolyn opted out of this one.

I grabbed the pill out of his hand, popped it into his mouth and tried to get him to lie down on the floor. Now, our bathroom is small, and with two stools, a four-year-old and a nine-year-old with her pants around her knees, a wife-mummy type and a chubby husband type, you can imagine the difficulty. Sarah somehow squeezed out and got a pillow and a large towel to cover Alan (because, you see, he was standing on his own towel), and I helped him lie down between and around two stools, a toilet and various corners. By the time we had accomplished all of this, the seizure had stopped. We all resumed our activities but poor Alan never finished his nice warm bath. We have yet to figure out what triggered that one.

Sarah has been told more about her dad's prognosis. She sees a school counsellor from time to time and had imagined, as kids do, a situation much worse than it is. She had learned that chemo only buys two weeks and so figured her dad had only two weeks to live. She didn't want to burden us with that, but fortunately she told the school counsellor, who asked Sarah's permission to tell us. Sarah agreed and now she knows just how sick Alan is and how little we can tell her about the future, but that it is for sure more than two weeks!

All the children's teachers were aware of the situation throughout Alan's illness. They were, without exception, a wonderful support for the children.

Perhaps it is the change that the tumour has brought to us, but Alan and I have started on some sort of clearing-out therapy. We've tossed incredible amounts of stuff out of closets and basement storage. For example, I had saved roughly 100 baby food jars in various sizes as well as six large cans of paint labelled "OLD – THIS COLOUR NO LONGER USED" and "USED 1983 ONLY." Alan still had his high school notes and so on. It's been wild to see just what we put in boxes and hid on shelves. I did keep 80 or so mason jars. Clearly, at some point in my life, I actually made pickles, jams and other preserves. With the change in the millennium coming perhaps I'll fill them this year. If you believe that...

Alan has had his first cup of real tea since about January 5, and the dietary restrictions lift on Wednesday for two weeks. He is already chilling the beer he will have Wednesday night. His appetite is fantastic, thanks to the steroids he is on to prevent swelling of the brain. The VON nurse asked whether he would like to see a nutritionist so I could make better meals. Alan said that I was doing just fine with the nutrition part but that he would have to stop at, say, three helpings rather than going onto five!

Since I last wrote, we have had the pleasure of stomach flu (Andrew and Carolyn), a badly strained foot (Andrew, needed X-rays), a sprained finger (Sarah), three bad throats (all the kids, and I'm getting that one now), and a badly bruised hip (Carolyn). I must say I love winter with all its injuries and germs. Alan has been saved thus far from the sore throat and the stomach flu, since he is not allowed to be kissed by sick kids or sick wives. Needless to say, holding buckets and cleaning up floors is off limits, too.

Chemo starts again in mid-February.

Moyra

Thursday February 4, 1999

We have had a setback of sorts in the last 24 hours. Alan has likely picked up strep throat from me, and I never even kissed him! Last night we had a great dinner, improved greatly by the surprise drop off of a bottle of fantastic foreign beer by one of our friends. Al enjoyed every sip of his half. I claimed the other half. There is no point overdoing things. He had a good evening, except for a mild seizure while sanding a few blocks of wood; that's the old left-right motion problem we've seen before.

At 2:00 a.m., Andrew got croupy and, before I got back to bed, Alan upchucked and missed the bucket – impressive! I drugged him with anti-nausea stuff and hoped for sleep. No such luck. By 7:00 a.m., Andrew was feeling much better – well enough to dump his toy box out all over his room looking for a particular toy. This woke Al, who proceeded to get flucus-of-the-tochus (diarrhea) big time and then spiked a high fever.

Once again, I tested the wonders of our health system and within minutes was talking to medical types and answering all kinds of questions. Alan had faded out of the picture and just lay on the couch looking grey. At that moment, the VON nurse arrived on the scene (early) and helped out. She did the blood-pressure type stuff and arranged for a lab technician to come to our house to take blood samples. At that point, the hospital called back and the doctors said, "Bring him in. He is likely neutrapenic." The VON told me this, and from his fever-sleep-greyness, Alan said, "What are they going to do with my penis?" I guess these things are important to guys!

In any case, neutrapenia is related to a low white blood cell count due to chemo, so off we went, my throat and Alan to "stretcher bay," which is not a southern resort. We were met by a neat team of nurses and a doctor and five hours later, after blood tests, X-rays, an IV and me pushing Alan around a hospital in a stretcher (to save time, since the porters were busy), he was sent home to sleep and will be stuffed with antibiotics over the next ten days.

Stay tuned. When he wakes up, I'm sure he is going to ask, "What did all of that have to do with my penis?"

We were humbled while we were at the hospital by a young couple with two children under five. The mum has metastatic cancer all over – she is maybe 35 – and the dad is holding it all together. Watching her tolerate the incredible pain was inspiring, to say the least.

Moyra

Monday, February 15, 1999

We've had the best week in about five months, once Alan recovered from whatever it was that caused the fever last week. As it turned out, he tested negative for strep. Likely, he had the kids' stomach flu. He has been sleeping better and generally has more energy. The children spent some really good time with him playing games and just talking.

On the seizure side, he is averaging about one per week at the moment. These we can control with the sublingual (under the tongue) Ativan. The neurologist detected some improvement in the level of intracranial pressure. He can now see a pulse in Alan's left eye. When the pressure is high (as it has been), the pulse is not present, since the blood flows but without the obvious pulse. Also, there is less drift of his left arm in the "hold out your arms with your eyes closed and hold them there for 30 seconds" test. Alan has also managed to reduce his steroid dose by one tablet a day. This also indicates a reduction in pressure. What we don't know is whether the pressure is going down because the radiation-related brain swelling is going down, or because the tumour is growing less actively or is maybe stalled in its growth, or a combination of the two factors. In any case, to have been able to reduce the steroid is a good thing. He is supposed to be completely off them by now but clearly that is not going to happen. He will just wean himself off them as soon as he is able.

Carolyn is sorting through the consequences of his illness in her own little mind. Andrew is handling it differently. He has announced that he is never going to move out and that he is going to stay with Mummy "forebber." I guess he is feeling quite concerned because when I had stomach flu last week and ached all over (I think a truck drove over me when I wasn't watching), Andrew just sat with me on the bed and watched television. Every now and again, he would ask whether I was going to be okay. Once he knew that it was just the same thing he had had the previous week and that soon I would stop throwing up, he seemed much more at ease, but still stayed very close to me. I gather from those of you with teenagers that there will come a time when I will be able to go to the bathroom and throw up in a private kind of misery, without small heads peering through the door wanting to know whether I am okay or offering to sit and "stay with you, Mummy."

Sarah becomes teary rather easily but seems to enjoy school, piano lessons, gymnastics and swimming. I am having to overcome mother-fear at gymnastics, since she is now doing rather scary moves such as front flips, front somersaults on the trampoline and front handsprings off the balance beam. I remind myself that she could have decided to take up juggling with sharp knives, or the local equivalent – hockey.

This week, we begin cycle two of chemo. Next week, we see the surgeon about a possible debulking (what an interesting word) of the tumour and the ramifications of that. We expect he will order an MRI so he can tell what part of the ugly stuff is related to radiation necrosis (dead tissue) and what is tumour. On a CT scan it is difficult to differentiate the two, but on an MRI I gather it is possible. So, when we know, I'll let you know.

Thanks for your Valentine's Day cards and wishes.

Moyra

Wednesday, February 17, 1999 – Alan, on the family dynamic

It has taken a week now to get back to where I was before that episode last week with the fever. The blood tests didn't show anything, so it was probably my turn for the flu that's been going around. I feel great now – hard to believe that anything is wrong. I just tire quickly and have memory problems. (So what else is new?) I'll take my good news where I find it.

Everybody here is working through the future possibilities in their own way. Carolyn and I were having breakfast together one morning last week when she said, "Daddy, it would be better for you to die first rather than Mummy because you would have your seizures and we couldn't drive the car so we would have to walk everywhere." It certainly raised my eyebrows! Just goes to show you that even at less than five years old they are absorbing more than we give them credit for and making use of the information in new ways that we have not spoken of. We'll have to pay attention to communication to ensure they don't get wrong ideas.

Andrew, like me, seems to be pretty much oblivious to what goes on that doesn't affect him directly. I'm sure he absorbs it, too, but talks less. Sarah has a counsellor at school to talk to, which helps her, no doubt, but again we'll have to talk to her more. She, too, is more stoic around us, so it's hard to say what she feels.

Returning to other matters, depression is much more common than most people understand. I have had it on and off for 20 years or more. Each cycle gets worse, but it's so easy to treat nowadays. At least I never spent a whole day lying on the floor unable to summon the strength to get up. The general population has a lazy/weak/selfish theory of the cause, but it's better not to listen to the a-holes on television and radio. It's no shame to need the medication. I wear glasses because my eyes don't work perfectly. Are diabetics lazy or weak because they take insulin?

The family is as you would expect. Moyra has her up and down times. The kiddies are very frightened by the possibility of more seizures, but now that my grouchiness has moderated they will sit next to me. Things are easiest for me. Since whatever the eventual outcome is doesn't trouble me, I can be passive and float along. It provides a better perspective on careers, work and material things, whatever.

Alan

Tuesday, February 2, 1999 – Alan, on faith, to Bob

In an earlier e-mail I may have ascribed to Aristotle the debating technique of asking questions until the opponent's argument falls apart. It was, of course, Socrates. I don't even recall what I said; deep-fried brain is all I can think of.

I'm afraid that your author returns to his lazy/weak/selfish theory of depression once too often. (Stand by for a mood swing.) It had me howling. If I had not been afraid of breaking something, I really would have thrown the book across the room. Like many experts, he has trouble keeping his opinions to subjects he knows something about. Now, in the face of abundant medical evidence going back over generations in some English families showing that depression has a genetic component, often associated with other problems or above-average intelligence, he has to advance this crackpot idea. It makes me suspect the quality of other arguments. How credible would people think him if he started arguing that disease was not caused by germs but was due to immoral habits? His kind of stupidity makes me furious. Worse than being wrong, his theory actually prevents people from seeking treatment.

I'll thank you for the book anyway. It was a kind and caring act. I am not, however, suffering. As an old-time pagan, I never needed an explanation for why things happen. Bad things happen sometimes. We all die some time. Could be a truck with your name on it, or buying a ticket on the wrong flight. With your tolerance, I won't read any more of this book.

Alan

Thursday, February 11, 1999 – Alan, on retirement

It's something of a relief now that all I have are self-imposed deadlines, meaning that since I don't have to earn anything I do only an hour or two of work a day. It's mainly for my amusement and to keep from going crazy from boredom. I don't recommend disability leave, but if you call it retirement it sounds a lot more fun. I had always had an ambition to become deadwood by 45 to get that golden handshake. If I'm not very careful all I'll achieve is the first half of that ambition, the dead part, and not the golden handshake. It may be that I'll get my golden handshake from St. Peter, no less.

I had no idea that the Teletubbies were spreading homosexual propaganda. Looking at their headgear, I saw two bottle openers and two corkscrews, obviously promoting alcohol consumption, plus all the colours of hangovers.

Alan

Wednesday, February 17, 1999 – Alan, with February blahs, to Janet

Maybe you remember (maybe you don't) what a difference the longer days make up here where the four seasons are Early Winter, Middle Winter, Late Winter and Next Winter, but that alone is enough to pick up anyone's mood. Of course, Ottawa has only has two seasons: winter and three months of tough sledding. Being outside is a pleasure now. You can really feel the power of the sun on your face, or anything else that's sticking out, but be careful. Getting sunburn and frostbite on the same body part is no fun.

Alan

Thursday, February 18, 1999 – Alan, ready for more chemotherapy

Having a (possibly) terminal illness changes attitudes towards everything. It's never just a headache anymore. If the weekly message gets missed, it's never just because of being forgetful or too busy. I'm sure Moyra appreciates having someone to download to. It's an awful burden for her. Doing all the housework is something she's had years of practice at, but

*all the child care plus the thought of widowhood at 45 (or sooner) makes
for a big load. I only have to go with the flow, an expression that takes
on new meaning if you have ever listened to lectures on sewer design.
Yes, civil engineers get whole courses on sewer design, and flow is what
goes through a sewer.*

*The second cycle of chemo starts today so no beer, no caffeine and no
old cheese for four weeks. Fortunately, sex is still allowed, and as with
most disabilities, you compensate by focusing on what you can do rather
than what you cannot.*

Alan

Many of our friends sent jokes by e-mail. Laughing truly is a good
therapy. This was one of the best jokes we received. I suppose it struck
a little too close to home in terms of our respective preferences, but
both Alan and I got a huge kick out of it. Intimacy was something we
still shared, as his e-mail above reveals. It allowed us to escape for a
little while from the day-to-day difficulties we faced.

THE PERFECT DAY FOR HER

8:15   Wake up to hugs and kisses

8:30   Weigh in five pounds lighter than yesterday

8:45   Breakfast in bed (fresh-squeezed orange juice and croissants)

9:15   Soothing hot bath with fragrant lilac bath oil

10:00   Light workout at club with handsome, funny personal trainer

10:30   Facial, manicure, shampoo and comb-out

12:00   Lunch with best friend at outdoor café

12:45   Notice ex-boyfriend's wife; she has gained 30 pounds

13:00   Shopping with friends, unlimited credit

15:00   Nap

16:00   Three dozen roses delivered by florist; card is signed "secret
admirer"

16:15   Light workout at the club, followed by gentle massage

17:30   Pick out outfit for dinner, primp before mirror

19:30   Candlelight dinner for two, followed by dancing

22:00   Hot shower (alone)

22:30   Make love

23:00   Pillow talk, light touching and cuddling

23:15   Fall asleep in his big strong arms

THE PERFECT DAY FOR HIM

6:00   Alarm

6:15   Sex

6:30   Massive dump while reading sports section of *USA Today*

6:40   Breakfast (filet mignon and eggs, toast and coffee)

7:00   Limo arrives

7:45   Bloody Mary en route to airport

8:15   Private jet to Augusta, Georgia

9:30   Limo to Augusta National Golf Club

9:45   Front nine at Augusta (two under)

11:45   Lunch (two dozen oysters on the half shell, three Heinekens)

12:15   Sex

12:30   Back nine at Augusta (four under)

14:15   Limo back to airport (Bombay Martini)

14:30   Private G4, Augusta to Nassau, Bahamas (nap)

15:15   Late-afternoon fishing excursion with all-female (topless) crew

16:30   Land world-record light-tackle Marlin (1,249 pounds)

17:00   Jet back; get massage and hand job en route

18:45   Shit, shower and shave

19:00   Watch CNN news flash: U.S. president resigns

19:30   Dinner (lobster appetizers, Dom Perignon [1963], 20-ounce New York steak)

21:00   Remy Martin and Cuban Partagas cigar

21:30   Sex

23:00   Massage and jacuzzi

23:45   Bed (alone)

23:50   Twelve-second, four-octave fart; dog leaves room

23:55   Giggle yourself to sleep

Monday, February 22, 1999

It has been another pretty good week for Alan. He is still averaging one focal/motor (hand- or leg-shaking) seizure a week but, so far, the Ativan (anti-seizure drug) has arrested them. His short-term memory seems to be improving, and his temper with the kids is steadily getting more and more normal. He has started reading them Winnie-the-Pooh in the evening. It is a real pleasure to see them snuggled up against him again. The second cycle of chemo is going well. He is less tired this time but had a bit more nausea in the early days of the cycle. He still has two good naps every day.

Today, we saw the neurosurgeon, who is in favour of a debulking surgery at some point. He has ordered an MRI to sort out what is tumour and what is necrotic (dead) tissue in the brain area. We finally saw Al's December 16 CT scan results and, although they were ugly, they weren't as bad as we expected they might be. By December 16, the bad area (tumour plus dead tissue) had regrown from the post-surgery size to more than half the size it was when Alan had the seizure in August. Clearly, it's a fast-growing SOB. That scan is now two months old. With luck, the chemo is working on this thing and buying time for Alan. Once we've seen the MRI, we will know whether a debulking operation is the way to go. In the meantime, we'll throw all the chemicals we can at it.

Carolyn has had a great week. She sheared the front off one baby tooth in a playground accident involving a game called battling, which the teachers have kindly banned, since it involves one kid throwing him/herself on the back of another in order to defeat the enemy. This also causes interesting bruises around the knees, elbows and facial area. So, off we went to the dentist to see about the survival rate of nerves in baby teeth. Just a few days later at my mother's, the same child had a collision with a sandstone wall and shoved her two front baby teeth through her lower lip while simultaneously pushing one of those front teeth up into the gums. Off we went again to the dentist (no stitches, but lots of swelling and bleeding). I got lots of neat stares at the store as I tried to explain in checkout lines that I didn't hit my child; she just walks into walls a lot. Anyway, now that the swelling has gone down we are getting X-rays to be sure there is no other damage to the nearby teeth. Of the three kids, Carolyn is the most like I was. She is a can't-sit-still, wiggly little thing who is always bruised and bashed. Let's hope her friends will do better than my friends, who foolishly followed me when I jumped out of trees (I got a bruised knee; my friend broke her leg) and across ditches (I skinned my elbow; my friend got stitches). Amazingly, they both still speak to me!

Sarah and Andrew keep a very close eye on Alan these days. If they find him in a different room from the special canister of Ativan, they will take it to him and say, "Daddy, you left this." The other day, Al was going to build a castle for Andrew and Andrew said, "Are you sure you should, Daddy? It might cause a seizure." It didn't this time, and I guess that is good, too.

So, we'll see how fast an MRI comes our way. We have learned that the faster these things happen, the sicker you are. A delay should be regarded as a good sign.

Moyra

Monday, March 1, 1999 – Alan to Janet

Aren't seizures just the most fun you can have by yourself? Luckily for me, the under-the-tongue Ativan is pretty good at stopping them cold, and I'm getting better at predicting when they are imminent. First, the strange out-of-body feeling 30 minutes beforehand, then the eyes flicking back and forth in the last 30 to 40 seconds. By then, it's time to drop everything, get the drug under the tongue and find the floor before it finds you! A loud "Oh shit!" helps when I want any company and Moyra is near enough to hear. Last week, I was in time to stop it before it got further than a twitching left hand. I was quite pleased by that success. But my overconfidence has caught me a couple of times. I finally found a doctor who would admit that being overtired helped bring on seizures. The others were only willing to admit to excess intracranial pressure and scrambled connections, dismissing my own experience, I guess, as anecdotal or the ravings of someone with obvious brain damage.

One of the forms I was asked to fill out was a family tree listing the number of people who had had cancer of one sort or another. Quite revealing. All I can say is that it is more than just the verbal diarrhea that has prevented any great writers from appearing in my ancestors. The colon cancer alone would be enough.

Alan

Wednesday, March 10, 1999

Six months have now passed since Alan was diagnosed with GBM. The news continues to knock us down. Somehow we pick ourselves up and continue. Today, we received the latest news about his MRI. An MRI gives better resolution than a CT scan. We had hoped (I prayed) to see that some of the size was radiation necrosis (dead tissue). It appears that it's all tumour. Worse, it is now the same size as at diagnosis although there is less pressure now than then. His brain midline is still straight, so he is not experiencing much effect on the left side, although he feels a bit weak. It is so hard to hug this big, strong person who seems to be so much himself and try to grasp the severity of the situation. The surgeon is prepared, based on Al's overall cognitive and physical abilities, to do the surgery again. He is going to talk to Al's medical and radiation oncologists to see what the best approach might be. For example, it might be a good time to put in glial wafers (local chemo) and to culture the cells to see what therapeutic chemo agents this thing might be susceptible to. There still might be benefits coming from the radiation. I have been told that it continues to do some work even now, but that it would have been a better sign if the tumour had responded to it more obviously. The benefits from chemo, if any, will not show until after the third cycle. We are almost at the end of cycle two.

Al is pretty discouraged today. He felt so strong last week and had told me he expected good news this time. He must be so disappointed. I think I knew it was coming. I saw some very long faces on the technicians last Thursday as they processed his scans. I had hoped it might be my overactive imagination, but no such luck.

In the next two weeks, Alan will try to decide what to do. I guess for him it is a decision to continue to fight hard and risk the further impairment and the long struggle back, knowing it is still a long shot at best, or making the decision to fight less hard. I know what I want, but at some point the call is his, not mine, to make.

The kiddies are fine for now. Sarah sometimes wakes up at night and asks me to turn on the television in our room so that she can hear something (other than the sounds in her imagination, I suppose), and Carolyn is struggling with it a bit, too. She told a few children in her class that her daddy had his head opened up to get out a cancer and they didn't believe her and called her a liar. She was mightily miffed by this, so I've told her to tell them they are silly-billies and she is, too, right. Andrew has become very close to me and very protective of all his stuffed animals. He needs them to reassure himself, I think, but he is very tender with them, especially the one who "has seizures" a lot. Some mornings I wake up with three children lying in bed with me and we are all cuddled together like a heap of puppies. Mummy puppy is usually stiff from sleeping over and around small pointy elbows and knees. Daddy puppy is in his own space in the single bed attached to the big one but even so, a leg, head or arm often strays into his territory.

Alan had a seizure at the dinner table the other day and, although he caught it early and it did arrest, he still ended up on the floor with kids getting blankets and pillows and me holding his head so it wouldn't rotate off. His head pulls around and he is powerless to stop it. Since it hurts like heck as it twists, I hold it back from this twisting and he is more comfortable. However, it is becoming a common enough occurrence that we seem, on the surface at least, to cope with it. I suppose the effects show up in our family cuddles and individual ways of sorting the problem out. Over the next few weeks, some more decisions will be made. Alan figures the positive side of hospitalization is the food. Sound backward? What he means is that he is looking forward to dropping some of his now more than 200 pounds as a result of dreadful food he will be fed while in hospital. His favourite meal last time was half a cold kid's meal pizza that we snuck in to him. The weight gain comes from the Decadron. It makes headaches go away but is a great appetite stimulant. We joke sometimes that his cup size is now much bigger than mine and I am getting jealous. On that note, I will paste a smile back on my face and continue one day at a time.

Moyra

Wednesday, March 10, 1999 – Alan thinks about surgery

As Moyra said, the surgeon is anxious to go ahead and carve some more tumour out. Personally, I would not at this stage if I were the only one involved. What I don't want to start is the "death by a thousand cuts," where a bit more is removed every six months or so until only a drooling idiot is left. I'm already close enough to that right now, thank you very much. More importantly, it has taken all this time from September to now to reach the point where I've recovered enough to realize what I have lost. As with any brain injury, the personality changes have left me grouchy, impatient and unpleasant enough that it's only in the last month that Andrew, Sarah and Carolyn will have anything to do with me. That, more than anything else, I don't want to lose again. Moyra keeps describing the choice as being one of continuing to fight on or deciding I've fought long enough, which is a dirty trick because she knows very well how I'd react to a choice like that. "Get me the f-ing knife. I'll do it myself."

You are right, however. I do tend to look at people, especially older ones that I don't particularly like, and ask why they get a long life, while I don't even get a decently long career. I still recall the people killed in that Swiss Air crash the same night I had my first surgery. They didn't even get six months to say goodbye.

Alan

As we approached the second surgery, I struggled with the futility of it all and sought advice from several sources. It was very challenging to find a balance between fighting the good fight and waving the flag of surrender. Ultimately, we chose life – which was still precious – knowing there were still things to try and still contributions to be made to both the family, mostly to the children, and to the science of understanding this disease.

Thursday, March 11, 1999 – from Dr. P. in Toronto

Thanks for keeping me informed. I understand your dilemma and you are not alone in wondering whether it is best to "go down fighting" or whether the treatments may be worse than the disease. Don't interpret a lack of shrinkage in the tumour as necessarily a bad thing. Of course, we would all like that to be the case, but no growth is still winning.

Dr. P.

Friday, March 12, 1999 – Alan, on bad news and reality

By now you should have been able to read Moyra's latest message, with all its bad news. Honestly, life is not supposed to be a race, but some people are so competitive they still have to be first across the finish line, even if there is no prize. To tell the truth, I had half expected bad news. My left arm and hand have been getting weaker and clumsier. My balance has been off a bit as well, so that whichever direction I walked felt like I was going downhill. The metaphor was not particularly attractive but in the end appropriate.

Since the beginning, the doctors have always been talking in terms of life extension only. I haven't believed them, being stubborn. I was going to be cured. Reality would behave as I said, not the other way around. As usual, the experts actually do know what they are taking about. So it may be that life extension and further surgery is the only game going. I'm not looking forward to becoming a drooling idiot but, being halfway there already, it's not that big a step. I'll let you choose which half.

Alan

Wednesday, March 24, 1999

We have been waiting for the surgeon, medical oncologist and radiation oncologist to have a chat about what is next for Alan. During the last two weeks, Alan was doing his part and deciding whether to have another craniotomy to remove the tumour. He is not looking forward to the surgery, but what really offends him is the idea of two weeks of eating at the hospital and being weak and helpless again. I pointed out that the Decadron had plumped him up a bit (he is about 210 pounds now), and two weeks of a strict, healthy, bland diet would be a bonus. After all, some people pay big bucks to be pampered on such diets at expensive spas. He agreed it might be the upside of the surgery.

Alan has made the choice to go ahead with another resection. On the one hand, it seems straightforward – buy time; on the other hand, it was a matter of "is fighting the good fight really worth it?" The medical types seem to take their cue from the patient. The more we ask, the more they seem willing to try to help us out.

During Alan's decision-making time, a number of interesting things happened. The children and I visited a pet store to pass the time one nasty winter afternoon and Sarah saw a poster for a colouring contest – win a free fish just for entering. I agreed (we have a tank), and one week later we had three fish. While waiting to get the fish we visited Toby, an African grey parrot who is very bright (she says hello and whistles at women). The little ones wanted to get Toby, too, but at $1,600, I said NO. Several more visits to the pet store have been required since then to feed Toby grapes. She loves them and the owner is happy to let Andrew and Carolyn feed Toby the most expensive type of seedless green grapes. Toby is a feather puller and on a strict controlled diet to help her feathers grow back. Green grapes are on her list. You can see what's coming can't you? But you are not quite right.

Sadly, Sarah's fish died last week and we went to the pet store again to replace the so-called free fish. While waiting, we visited Toby. All three kids were so sad. I guess we all feel that Toby's condition can be cured, and we so much want to cure something – anything. Just then I heard a whistle behind me and there, on top of its cage, was a beautiful cockatiel.

Now, I am not a bird person (except in feeders outside), and we have a cat (albeit very old, nineteen, and somewhat demented). At that point, the staff member put the bird on my finger and that was it. The kids were enthralled. The bird crawled up my arm and onto my shoulder and began to nibble my ear. Then the staff member gave the bird to Sarah and in turn to the other two kids, and within two minutes the bird had a name and I wasn't saying no very hard. After all, the social workers say a lot about building memories and making happy times.

I called a halt to things and offered them McDonald's for dinner, hoping perhaps to deflect their combined interest. Not a chance. Three little angels did the eye-batting, promise-to-clean-the-cage, he's-so-cute routine that thousands of other parents have fallen victim to, and I was no exception. So, I set the maximum price firmly on the table and off we went to pick up the bird. I'm a softie, because when that bird started to hop up and down when he saw us again I was a goner. I asked the staff if it was a boy or girl. Since the bird is so young it's too early to say, but if it sings a lot, it's a boy. Needless to say, the starter kit cage was too small for this three-month-old cockatiel, and my firmly set price was not as firm as I thought, since the children insisted on adding the necessary toys to his cage, including Andrew's choice of a $14 bell.

Perky is now a member of the family. The cat can't believe his aging eyes and thinks he is hallucinating. I am not all that confident that Perky won't end up as the dinnertime treat of the year. Perky acts like a small, feathered child or husband that sings to me when I enter the room and nibbles my ears. He is happiest when out of the cage enjoying the family. He sat on Sarah's shoulder last night, bobbing up and down as she practised the piano.

To my surprise, Alan has taken to this creature and is teaching the bird to make a two-tone whistle. They have lunch together when I'm at the office, and Alan has had lots of fun rearranging the perches in the cage and building a portable perch. It is giving him something to do that is kind of pleasant. Since the two of them rise with the sun, they keep each other company. The last few days have been a bit brighter and cheerier as we marvel at this little creature with a brain the size of a pea that has already learned the commands "up" (on the finger), and "stay" (when he wants to fly off his cage). Oddly enough, this cheerfulness seemed to help Alan come to terms with his decision to go ahead with the surgery.

The focus on a new life in our family was wonderful. There was something refreshing and delightful about it that counterbalanced Alan's illness. Both Alan and I grew up with pets and enjoyed the companionship they provided. Even our grumpy old cat, Sandy, added a certain flavour to the household. The presence of our pets, their unconditional love and all their antics came to be a substantial comfort for us. I was fully aware that I would be the one who did the majority of the additional work and, in the back of my mind, I worried that we might have to cope with an illness or the death of a pet. Still, at that time, the joy introduced by a little bird far outweighed any other concerns.

The meeting with the doctor this morning was fascinating. He outlined the next set of possibilities. We are going to try to follow the protocol to get a fresh section of the tumour for the folks in Edmonton who are doing reovirus phase two testing, and we might get another piece for chemo-therapeutic testing of the tissue for sensitivity to various chemo drugs. (This is less certain, since, most of the time, the clinician's experience is as good as anything else.) There is the possibility now of going to the U.S. for gamma knife radiation treatment (there are five gamma knives in the U.S., and none in Canada at this point) after surgery but we're told there is now a phase two trial in Ottawa on the Canadian version of a gamma knife.

I gather the gamma knife radiation treatment machine is costly. Canadians and most U.S. centres use the existing equipment to do focused stere-otactic radiation, which mimics the gamma knife and is, I gather, just as good. Since Alan is at his lifetime limit for radiation to the brain, this focused-beam technology is really neat. Instead of three big beams passing through the brain and damaging good tissue as well as tumour tissue, the focused therapy works by having many little beams of a very small dose focused on the same spot – right smack dab in the middle of the tumour, significantly reducing the exposure of the rest of the brain to the radiation. So, after this resection, we will wait for the healing and then go back to more radiation this special way. Does it work? Like most of these studies, there just aren't enough people with this kind of disease to tell. The short answer is probably not, but it should buy more time to try something else.

The reovirus testing, for example, requires two months for the reovirus to infect the fresh tissue in the lab. Next, it has to be tested for toxicity and then put back into the patient's brain in the hopes that it will infect the rest of the growing tumour. We hope we can get in line for that, too. We are not sure what happens about the chemo treatments. Alan's third cycle is set to go on April 1. I would like him to get the third cycle under his belt, since chemo involves a systemic poison and will get to the parts of the brain where stray tumour cells are sitting waiting and thinking about making colonies. At the moment, the MRI shows no obvious tendrils of tumour or new sites, which is part of the reason Alan can have surgery again.

He is feeling a bit better this week, although his left side is clearly weaker than it was even last week. The left-side weakness causes him to leave his arm behind. For example, a few days ago he found his hand tucked neatly under his belt, where he had been stuffing his shirt into his pants. It's a bit like the electrical lines are down. I sometimes have to remind him to use his left arm while he is eating. We have increased his Decadron back to where it was a month ago to help reduce the pressure inside his skull, which is likely causing these problems.

I think, having made the decision to do the surgery, he now wants to get it over with. I'll send another e-mail out in a few weeks when we know more. At the moment, surgery is scheduled for April 13.

Moyra

Wednesday, March 31, 1999 – Happy Easter 1999

The sun is shining here, and Alan is feeling as well as he has in a few weeks. He is not looking forward to surgery but is fairly resigned to giving it a try. He had a humdinger of a seizure earlier this week. It was so bad that he asked me to hold him down. Fortunately, he stayed conscious and there wasn't much residual paralysis. I went, in a matter of moments, from preparing a lecture on statistical process control and 6-sigma quality at one end of the dining table, to dropping meds in his mouth and holding down his arms and legs at the other end. After that, I vowed I would never again complain about having to prepare new lecture material.

Alan was quite amused when the surgeon's nurse called the other day and scheduled a pre-operative appointment for April 20. Alan asked if this was a new approach, to have the pre-operative appointment seven days post-operative. There was a long pause on the other end and the nurse said something like, "Ah, well, I'll have to get back to you on that." Chemotherapy has been postponed for now. Alan was to start cycle three tomorrow, but the medical oncologist thought Alan should get back his strength a bit before surgery. This means that he can have a beer or two before surgery – maybe even a scotch.

This is the weekend of the cakes, so Alan is mustering his strength for Andrew and Carolyn's fifth birthday party for their friends, the birthday party for the family and the arrival of the Easter bunny. I call it the weekend of the cakes because I make four birthday cakes: one shared for school, two for the kids' party and one, if I have any energy left, for the family. I always hope there will be leftovers.

For those of you who asked, Perky the bird is still alive, although Sandy the cat is now pretending to sleep under the dinner table waiting for Perky to have a bad landing. The bird can fly across the room but has trouble developing lift. For you aero-types, he develops quite nice drag. As a result, it is more of a well-controlled crash than a true flight. His flight feathers are slightly clipped, so it must be a challenge to get into the air at all. Perky loves to take showers in the sink and displays his wings when he wants the kids to fly him. He accompanied Sarah into the bathroom the other day and nearly fell-flew into the tub so I guess that is out for a while. He has said his first word: "hello" in bird baby talk. Like all youngsters, his voice is still underdeveloped but his screeches are not. The children are enchanted.

I think the bird wonders what he did to be tormented (albeit lovingly) by three children and a quite clearly demented adult female (me) who pesters him incessantly, saying, "Hello, hello, hello" over and over again. I don't want yet another creature saying, "Mummy, Mummy, Mummy," so I am teaching it the word *hello*. I'm not entirely sure what Alan is teaching the bird. They have an early breakfast together each morning and I hear them chatting. I am quite sure I'll know what expression came from Alan when Perky first shares it with me.

Moyra

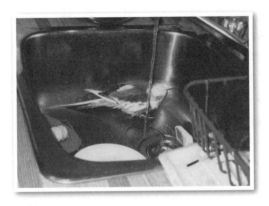

PERKY ENJOYS A SHOWER IN THE KITCHEN SINK.

Thursday, April 13, 1999

Well, the bad dream continues, as we faced round two of surgery today. As you know, Alan has not been looking forward to this but was in good spirits yesterday as he went in. He flirted (as nicely as a guy can when his wife is with him) with the lady nurses, had a good dinner, but complained about the lack of gravy, and even shaved this morning.

He did the blood workup stuff last night. I gave the nurses his list of medications and the variations with each meal and they did their best to keep it straight. In the end, I made them repeat it back to me to be really sure and, yes, they made one small error. One of the nurses asked me to describe the seizures, and when I was done she was quite impressed with our calmness.

This morning at 6:00 a.m. I went over to the hospital and stayed with him past the "authorized people only" sign. The staff let me go there last time, too, but you have to smile and promise to keep quiet. The nursing staff is fantastic. As we waited, there were four operating theatres going.

Alan and another man discussed the relative merits of their respective surgeries. Both wanted to be elsewhere and both expected four hours under, but the other guy had these nice white pressure stockings on – he was in for a prostate removal. He and Al agreed that the doctors could do anything as long as it worked afterward. I reminded Al of that an hour or so ago when I visited him in the special observation unit. He looked me straight in the eye and said it would probably kill him to even try.

When I left, Alan was worried about having another seizure – he felt weird. But one does, I guess, when one has tubes running in and out all over the place. With the tumour gone again, he ought to be free of seizures for a while, as long as his anti-seizure drug levels are therapeutic.

The tumour was every bit as big as it was six months ago. The size, a drink of wine and a late dose of medication probably explain the terrible seizure Alan had at 3:00 in the morning the night before heading into hospital. It was his first night-time seizure, but he managed to get the pill in his mouth before shouting at me that he would need help. It was a really bad one and he needed three pills before it began to arrest. This tumour doesn't give us any relief from its growth.

Alan is quite uncomfortable at the moment and has told me, "I'm not doing this again!" As you can see, there has been no cognitive decline, as far as I can tell, at least and so far, touch wood, no paralysis. He can't walk or anything like that yet, but he might be allowed to sit up tomorrow.

I am very grateful to have Perky the bird around. He is, as one friend put it, a healthy distraction. He is very friendly and has won over both grandmothers. He sits happily on their shoulders when they visit. The kids love him to bits and Sarah spends a lot of time just stroking his head and talking to him softly. Perky is a good listener and I think it helps her deal with Al's situation. Perky talks most to Sarah. I think he admires her long blonde ponytail, as in, "Look at the feathers on that one – nibble, nibble, coo."

Perky is most cuddly with Andrew and likes to tuck his head under Andrew's chin. Perky is a bit puzzled by Carolyn, as she likes to have Perky on her shoulder when she brushes her teeth. Perky looks with considerable confusion at the electric toothbrush, staring out one side of his head and then the other at this noisy white thing. On several occasions now, Perky has joined the kids in the bath. The first time was by accident, but now he sits on their legs, up to his tummy, having a grand time. It is such a hoot. Alan refers to Perky as my second husband: he nibbles my ear and needs lots of TLC but at least can be put in a cage when he is annoying.

As the monitors ground on today and I watched Al's heartbeat and respiration rate and all that stuff, I was struck by the amount of equipment and the impersonalness of it all. Tubes and lines and monitors all over. Still, by tonight, he was off oxygen and by tomorrow he should be off most of the monitors. The nurses check on him very often, since he is in a special observation unit. As I said, they are uniformly wonderful and do their best to reassure all the patients there. It's funny how one learns to share knowledge and coping strategies. Several strangers who were experienced with the routines of the neuro-observation area helped me when Al was first diagnosed. Total strangers become quite close and share the ups and downs. Today, I spent a lot of time (while I waited for Alan) talking to the family of a man who had just arrived, explaining how the place worked.

If anything interesting happens, I'll send out some news. Otherwise, a few weeks in hospital and then Alan returns home.

Moyra

In the very beginning, we had asked the doctors to be completely open with us with respect to diagnosis, pathology and prognosis. After Alan's first surgery, I had delayed giving Alan all the details, although he knew the basics, since we wanted to give him a bit of a chance to heal physically.

That delay caused a problem after his second surgery. Alan was convinced I was hiding something and, although he had already seen the scan clearly showing one large tumour, he came to believe he had multiple large tumours. Of course, he didn't. This marked a bit of a turning point, since clearly he didn't trust me to tell him the truth and he didn't trust the nurses, either. In some ways, he was being consistent, since he believed in Alan. I had to ask his surgeon to explain how the surgery had gone. Thankfully, Alan believed the surgeon, the local scientific authority. After that incident, I put everything back on the table and we continued to ask for all the details all the time.

Nevertheless, there was a point late in his illness at which Alan simply stopped asking for information. I knew by then that people tend to either want all the information or very little of it. Alan seemed to have moved into the second group. Perhaps it was simply too much to bear. I took that as my cue and began to receive some of the information on my own. When he asked, I did my best to explain as honestly and gently as I could.

Friday, April 14, 1999

To my amazement, and with some help, Alan got up and walked around the neuro-observation unit this morning. He is doing so very well. Better than last time; of course, he was healthier starting out this time. All the tubes and drains are out. All the concern over his peculiar heartbeat signature that was registered by his arterial line (yup, in the artery) was resolved, too. Someone had put two leads on the left and one on the right (or vice versa) instead of two on the right and one on the left (or vice versa). In any case, it made his heartbeat waveform strange, and there was some puzzlement over that.

His left hand is twitching constantly, so his drug levels are being raised again. The hope is that it is caused by swelling in the brain (edema). Al hates the twitching because it feels like a seizure is about to happen. It isn't, but it feels that way. The pharmacology expert dropped by to chat about Alan's drugs. She was a very cheerful sort. She suggested he move to 5 g each day (he is on 2.5 g) of one of his medications. In the end, we decided to up it bit by bit until his hand stops shaking.

It's been a good day in many respects, although Alan is very depressed this time around. Last time, he didn't really believe the diagnosis. This time I think he does, at least for the moment. But, knowing Alan, in a few days he'll be all set for the thing guys like most in the world.

To treat myself, after doing some marking today, I had a facial. Wow. I should have done that years ago. The massage at the end of the facial was worth every penny. I nearly fell asleep on the table. That helped make up for the lack of sleep last night.

Once again, your support is a big help.

Moyra

Wednesday, April 19, 1999

Alan's recovery has gone quite well and he is now home in bed. He is able to walk on his own and is feeling a bit more upbeat than a few days ago. His left arm is quite twitchy still, with epilepsy-like behaviour in that arm. (An electroencephalogram showed he had brain waves consistent with those of epilepsy.) He has some more drugs to take to control the twitches. We hope that as the brain swelling from surgery goes down, the twitching will ease up, too, but there are no guarantees.

We learned that the radiation did have some effect on the tumour. The blood vessels around it were blocked (thrombosis) likely as a result of the radiation, so it appears that it did indeed slow the tumour's growth down a bit. We have been told that the tumour behaviour on regrowth can be quite different than during first growth and tends to be unpredictable. I hope to get more pathology stuff when Alan has his 27 staples removed in two weeks.

Perky nearly ended up in surgery this morning. Sandy, the cat, was sound asleep in the deep sleep of the elderly. Carolyn carried Perky to the bathroom to brush her teeth. Perky, in the wisdom of a pea-brained creature, decided to have a fly and flew right onto Sandy. Sandy might be elderly, but if you land on his back he is bound to take a swipe or two. Perky left a trail of tiny feathers on his second flight. I don't think Sandy tried very hard; I suspect he was insulted more than anything.

So, here we go on round two of radiation and new drugs and all the fun. Thanks for your support over the last week. I took all the e-mails in to Alan. He said that so many of you said, "Keep it up," that he wanted you all to be clear that Viagra is not one of the drugs he takes. As you can see, his peculiar sense of humour is intact.

Moyra

The results from Al's pathology after the second resection clearly showed that the radiation had been somewhat effective in stalling the tumour. We wondered what would have happened if Alan had not had the radiation and chemotherapy, since the tumour had continued to grow under both. However, there was never a moment of relief from the worry, since the pathology clearly indicated that, with anaplastic astrocytoma (a somewhat less aggressive brain cancer) and glioblastoma multiforme, the tumour was likely to return. We had more to come and very little time before it would begin growing again.

COMMENT: Sections of all specimens show the characteristic changes found in radiation necrosis including the development of large multinucleated giant cells with bizarre, irregular and hyperchromatic nuclei with some breakdown of their chromatin. To be noted as well was the severe decrease or absence of mitotic figures. It is impossible to tell with certainty that this tumor will not recur. Most observers are in agreement that with anaplastic astrocytomas and glioblastomas the tumor even though severely damaged by radiation in its center, often resumes growth about its periphery and often at an accelerated pace within 6 to 12 months after the maximum permissible radiation dose.

Wednesday, April 29, 1999

The sun is shining and Alan is enjoying the garden, grumbling about his draggy left arm and leg, and we are all smiling about his latest pathology. He had the 27 stainless steel staples removed on Tuesday and the healing was good. His pathology arrived by fax this morning. There is a wonderful neurology nurse cum community relations person at the hospital and she is so good to us.

It appears that the tumour was severely damaged by the radiation. The regrowth was a grade 2 and a grade 3 rather than the original level four. The mitotic figure rate is way down in some parts of the resection and was absent in other parts. This means the cell division is much slower in some spots and not present in others.

On the downside, the pathology also indicates that regrowth will resume about the periphery at an accelerated pace. We hope that additional radiation with the focused beam will help out there.

There is also a newer chemotherapy possibility – Temodal. This drug has been around for about 40 years in various forms, but the testing has recently passed from the monkey stage into human phase one and two trials and is now in phase three testing. It has come to market in Europe and is available in the U.S. on an experimental basis. It appears to be most effective on Al's type of tumour.

I gave Alan a bit of a haircut in the hospital because the one shaved side looked weird compared to the fluffy-sticking-up-grey-brown side. The shaved stuff is growing in quite nicely and he looks so much better without the zipper-head effect.

Alan is still struggling a bit with his weak left side. For the first week he was home, we covered some old territory as in, "Dear, could you do up my fly again and tie my shoes and button my cuffs?" Just for fun, try doing up your spouse's fly. It's not as easy at it appears, especially when the spouse in question is a guy and makes all kinds of wisecracks. In the end, I learned to stand behind him (it's safer there), reach around his Decadron tummy and pull up the zip. Elastic laces like the children wear have helped with the shoes. I toyed with the idea of yellow polka-dot laces but settled on black. Recently, I found Al walking around with his left hand stuck down the front of his pants. We all had a good laugh about it (it was just stuck there from tucking his shirt in).

Perky the bird continues to be an inspiration to us all. To my amazement, the other day he spoke again. I had given Alan something to eat and Perky was watching from the top of his cage. Alan did not remember to say the magic words, but out of Perky's beak came "Thank you." It's nice to know that someone is listening to my lectures on table manners.

Perky only says "hello" when he is very mellow and someone is stroking his neck. Come to think of it, Alan behaves similarly in the same situation. Perky is learning to rub his beak on someone's cheek when he hears "kiss, kiss." This is a real charmer for the kiddies, but for the moment Perky prefers to kiss me over all the others, although he clearly thinks Sarah's ponytail is the best in the family and likes to hide in and around it. While Alan was in hospital, Perky flew down from the cage and ran across Carolyn's plate, scattering scrambled eggs all over the place. She was quite miffed.

Since the last surgery, Alan's voice is very flat and emotionless, although it is slowly improving. The kids are having a bit of problem with this, as am I. The other day I had to ask him how he intended a particular comment, because it was a rather complex double entendre. When I explained the two meanings he clarified that it was meant to be self-deprecating, not insulting to me. It is a bit hard on visitors, too, since they don't know about the monotone voice. Alan has always been sort of deadpan and sarcastic in his joke telling, but with the latest change in voice his jokes don't sound like jokes at all. Yesterday I had to tell one of Alan's friends that Alan was joking about something. He thought Al was absolutely serious. So, be warned.

Moyra

3

May to December 1999

STEREOTACTIC RADIATION AND EXPERIMENTAL TRIAL

We discussed the various options with Alan's doctors and it seemed that the best next steps, after surgery, would be stereotactic radiation followed by second-line chemotherapy through an experimental trial. There was, for both of us, a desire to continue to contribute to the science of Alan's disease in a general sense and to gain knowledge for the extended family. Simply put, we continued our very active fight against the progression of the disease.

We had high hopes for the stereotactic radiation, since the pathology from the second resection had shown the first round of radiation had indeed affected the tumour. Participating in the experimental trial of a new chemotherapy meant signing a document in which Alan had to agree that his condition could not be cured by any standard treatment. I was now accustomed to seeing the word incurable; nevertheless, it continued to evoke a strong and unpleasant physical reaction.

I hoped the combination of the two treatments would buy us some quality time. Of course, we had no idea how much time it would buy nor if it would be quality time, but Alan always felt better when he was actively fighting the battle, and I thought it was a battle worth fighting.

Monday, May 3, 1999

We had a nice day at the lake, except Alan is really ticked at not being able to do what he wants, due to aching legs and weakness. It really bugs him that he cannot do what he wants to, when he wants to, and it's very stressful on all of us, especially when I tell him I want to know where he is going so I know where to look. He feels like I am treating him like a child, and I guess I am, in some respects, but when he wanders off for a walk around the block and doesn't tell me I find it a little freaky. Sigh – there is no way out of this one.

Sarah and I went for a swim at the lake – it was cold! – but I was so hot from all the work. At one point I was hanging out a window, Alan's arm around me, banging on a piece of vinyl siding to get it back in place. I resorted to a nail. It stays put now.

Moyra

Monday, May 17, 1999

Alan's recovery from the resection on April 13 is continuing. He feels stronger most days but still sleeps a lot – two or three naps per day, one to two hours each. Why so tired? Well, it could be the Frisium, which was added after the surgery as a further anti-convulsant. (It is very Valium-like in chemistry.) It could be normal post-operative recovery or it could be the continued progression of the illness. He had an MRI today that should give us more data. We are told that there are three possibilities. First, the tumour is gone and won't be back for a while (we hope for this). Second, the tumour is growing back in neat round nodules (we expect this) so that stereotactic radiation (radio-surgery) can be done later this month. Third, the tumour is growing back all over the surgical cavity (I pray against this), in which case we try chemo again and heaven only knows what else after that. In terms of recovery, Alan no longer needs me to do up his fly or his jacket, which is just as well. His short-term memory is brutal to deal with – I have to follow him around the house turning off taps, shutting drawers and closets, and putting lids on things. We almost had a bad accident at the lake on the weekend when he left the camp stove on, thinking it was off. So, no more propane, no camp fuel and no stoves for Alan.

As many of you know, Alan is very particular about his campfires. I'm afraid he was critical of mine at the lake, but with his balance and memory problems I figured no open fires, either. The trip to the cabin was so nice. We stayed over for the first time. It was built last fall when Alan was up to his eyeballs in surgery and was supposed to help out but was unable. Al's brother-in-law and the brother-in-law's father did it all.

I installed my first screen door, since Alan couldn't do it, although he helped manage. It was quite funny because the opening ended up being narrower and shorter than the closest standard. I bought a saw and manually removed the extra bit at the bottom of the door. Naturally, the generator and circular saw I would have liked to have used were at home. Getting the hinges under the vinyl siding was kind of fun, too. We decided that next time we build a cabin, the screen door goes in during building, not a year later. Fortunately, we had lots of bandaids, since the hinges, saw, screwdriver (Phillips, of course; why doesn't everyone use Robertson?) and siding all removed small pieces from my tiny fingers.

Actually, all this mechanical engineering stuff has come in handy this last year. I have installed new taps in several bathrooms and wrestled with the snow blower this winter. I have determined that Alan was right all along; snow blowers do work better when you swear at them. On the way to the lake, Alan had a nap in the car, so when we arrived he went off with Andrew to explore. Andrew's first words were, "Little weasel, I'm back." (Last fall, a weasel moved into the woodpile.) Andrew is clearly a woodsman and was off climbing trees and wandering around in the bush covered, but not bothered by, blood-sucking, voracious insects. (Carolyn puffs up like crazy.) However, when one of these fully loaded mosquitoes drowned in Andrew's milk he freaked out as blood oozed into the glass. I spent the next ten minutes trying to find a cup with a lid that no bug could fit through. Carolyn offered the suggestion that Andrew ought to stay in the umbrella gazebo where the bugs weren't. Sarah actually called the loons over so they were close to the shore. We hope they'll nest in our little bay.

We nearly gained a cat thanks to Andrew, too. He brought one over from the neighbours to visit us. The little stray was very affectionate, purred like crazy and sat on all the kids' laps. The neighbourhood news was that this cat had been left behind during a medical student move. I resisted for five days. We fed him outside, since the little hunter attempted to gain access to Perky the hand-fed bird. Sarah found out he answered to the name Ginger. One morning I took Ginger to the Humane Society but promised to retrieve him, if necessary. Thank heaven someone claimed him after only 24 hours. I think he must have been micro-chipped. So we are still a family of five humans, one elderly cat and a bird.

While we were at the MRI today, a young fellow sat down beside us. He was recently diagnosed with a form of sarcoma in his foot, and it had spread to his lungs. He is 27 and apparently for three years has had his foot pain misdiagnosed. Poor guy. It's funny how in a Cancer Centre we can share so much with total strangers. I guess it makes a common bond that is safe. You know the person next to you is in trouble, too, so out it all comes. There is a vulnerability that comes with serious illness but there is a hidden strength, too. Perhaps this is why so many of the wonderful volunteers at the Cancer Centre are survivors.

If all is as expected, Alan will have the stereotactic radiation on May 26. It's an all-day thing, starting with a stereotactic head frame that is screwed into Alan's skull at 8:15 a.m. and that he wears all day. CT scans and mapping of the tumour by radiation physicists follow, and then they blast the suckers. It takes about 45 minutes per nodule, I think. They try up to three or four nodules, as long as they are smaller than 3 cm in diameter.

I hope that is enough news for now. We are hanging in there and trying to be normal. I went to Sarah's school to teach sprinting last week and was pleased to find out I can still outrun all the Grade 4s. I suspect I am a lot stiffer this week, though, than they are.

Moyra

Wednesday, May 26, 1999

Alan's sense of humour is as keen as ever. He offers the following experience from our long weekend at the lake. He wants you to laugh, not cry.

BOATING WITH BRAIN DAMAGE

by Alan

I'm still learning what is gone and what remains. Some things I have outright lost completely; others are sort of remembered, but my coordination and balance are poor, making it exciting sometimes to do things like climb a ladder or walk down a set of rough stone steps. The three-dimensional mental manipulations, such as found in a lot of carpentry or wood butchery, are gone. I learned another this weekend. First, I want to emphasize that I have been messing about in boats since about the age of ten.

On the weekend I decided to take our very small rowboat out by myself. [He didn't tell me he was going to. – Moyra] *I stepped into the boat expecting to glide away from the dock, which it did until the rope I had forgotten to untie ran out of slack and the whole affair came to a sudden stop. I got pitched headlong into the bottom of the boat so my head was in the bottom and my feet were in the air over one gunwale. The whole boat was canted over at about 40 degrees and came close to capsizing from the unbalanced weight. I had to reach back behind my head to grasp the other gunwale and do what amounted to a push-up with my hands on one side of the boat and my legs sticking out over the other.*

When the rocking had subsided, I crawled into the boat and sat up, quite pleased that the whole thing had not gone over. That was when I heard the putt-putt of a boatload of fishermen going by. Oh well, you can't impress everybody, I guess.

BOATING SAFETY RULES. RULE #1: UNTIE THE BLOODY BOAT – it works a lot better that way.

Fortunately, Sarah had given him a life jacket.

The cabin is coming along nicely. At the end of the weekend, Alan remarked in surprise, "You're quite handy with tools!" I replied that I have always been handy with tools; he had just never noticed before. Mind you, it's tricky cutting quarter-round while simultaneously slapping mosquitoes and admiring the half-eaten fish head that nature boy (Andrew) is carrying. This time, I took along a brand-new first aid kit.

Today, Alan is in the hospital for his stereotactic radiation (also called stereotactic radio surgery). He is quite a sight with a piece of steel (I think) about 1 cm by 1 cm wrapped around his head and held up by four posts screwed into his skull. The ring of steel is at about eye level. He should be out of the gizmo within a few hours. The tumour, as we thought, is growing again. It is an irregular shape, a bit cone-like and back to about 2.5 cm along the long part of the cone. The rest of the cavity is clear, which is why he can have this procedure. The tumour has grown deeper and towards the ventricle (the ventricle contains cerebrospinal fluid), which is where the surgeon had to stop. Alan is quite cheerful, although not all that pleased to be in a head vise. He said that this was as close as he was ever going to get to wearing a halo.

Tomorrow (May 27) marks the day that I was told Alan might live to. He will pass the median survival rate for his illness. To me, it is pretty special. I will never forget the look on the surgeon's face when he said, "Nine months." It has been nine months in which we have had far too many lows and not enough highs – when the value of your friendship has held us together, when total strangers have given comfort by sharing their experiences. I don't know where we go from here, except we have learned to live a bit more in the present and not so much in the "someday when there is time I will…"

Moyra

The growth rate of GBM tumours is one of their most devastating characteristics. Alan's resection was excellent. Even so, after six weeks the tumour was back and had grown to 2.5 cm. Although we had seen this kind of growth rate after the original resection, we had hoped that the damage caused to the tumour by radiation and chemotherapy would have slowed the growth rate somewhat. We had hoped that we might be given half of the six months referred to in the pathology report after his surgery. Unfortunately, this was not the case.

Thursday, May 27, 1999 – Alan, on retirement

Yup, my vote is for early retirement. If there is any place you want to see, any toy you want to play with, now is the time to do it. Like everything, there are two problems to overcome. The first is, as always, money. My disability insurance only runs for two years. Putting it starkly, I have two years to get better or die. The second problem is one faced by most retirees: what the blazes do you do with each day? Did you ever see the movie The Shining? Not an ideal thing for people contemplating a long period of isolation. I have a workshop to butcher wood in and gardens to tramp around. I can do this in between naps and help Moyra with her research if any time remains.

As long as there is not too much cognitive damage, I expect I will continue with surgery. After all, I can still enjoy my children, even if boating is more of a challenge than it was. Besides, miracles happen every day. I have now beaten the average survival; its time to go for the gusto, as the Americans say.

Don't worry about what to write. Just knowing someone who cares is listening is a help. Attitude is everything in this game, I'm told.

Alan

Friday, May 28, 1999 – Alan, on stereotactic radiation

First, I want to thank you all for your messages of support; they are generally the highlight of my day. The tremor in my left hand is somewhat better now that I'm taking another anti-epileptic drug, although I now sleep an hour in the a.m. and two in the p.m. It makes getting anything done a bit slow. Two days ago I was back in the hospital for what is called stereotactic radiation – much narrower, more intense beams of X-rays are arranged to intersect at the tumour. It means they have to first bolt this crown to my head, make a CT scan to get the tumour coordinates and then transfer it all downstairs to the other machine before blasting away.

It's damned uncomfortable. The only amusement was to thrill the nurses with my Star Wars imitation: "LUKE, BEWARE THE DARK SIDE." They always laugh; they had probably only heard it 100 times that day.

Alan

Monday, June 4, 1999

Alan is sawing logs upstairs in the chair I bought for nursing the twins five years ago. Oddly enough, I've hardly ever used it, even when I was nursing. Alan likes it a lot. Perky the bird is nibbling Alan's buttons and marching up and down his chest, and seems to like the snores. Perhaps Perky will give us his rendition of snoring in future.

Today, we had back-to-back visits to the surgeon and medical oncologist. The surgeon has suggested we figure out a relationship between blood flow in the brain and waveform. It was very strange. I think he likes the fact that we know math. He often chats about his work. It is really quite nice.

My hope for using a newish release of the chemo drug Temodal, which we first learned about in April, was clobbered by the realization that Temodal works less well on those who have had CC (also called Lomustine), and since the C in Alan's PCV (procarbazine, CCNU and vincristine) was actually CCNU ... well, anyway, we were offered a couple more ideas.

The surgeon may digitize the CT scans and send them off to the Alberta gene therapy guy. Perhaps there is some hope there for the future. Also, the medical oncologist has a new trial on. The new trial works on the assumption that the blood brain barrier (BBB) has been disturbed big time by two resections, radiation and stereotactic radiation. So it means that more standard, but really good, chemo drugs might get by the BBB now.

I forgot to ask the oncologist how many of the people in his trial are still alive. There have been ten in the brain tumour part. Al will make eleven. On the upside, the tumour is as small as it has ever been. It stood at about 2.5 cm before the stereotactic radiation and we have another scan in two weeks.

The advantage of a clinical trial is lots of medical attention at all times. with doctors, nurses and triage types available. They seem to find it embarrassing when trial patients have bad reactions. We're not in a double-blind trial and we are changing drugs big time to more common chemotherapy drugs. I've never liked double-blind trials for terminally ill people. It's like saying, "You have a 50/50 chance of getting a placebo or something we think might work."

It's been exciting on the home front, too. I lost my wallet and discovered that one can recreate one's existence simply with a Zellers card and a photo from work. This allowed me to get my driver's licence. With a driver's licence and a passport, I managed to get my health card. So, I'm alive in the land of cards again. The wallet turned up after three days, the money gone and all cards moved, but back. New versions of all my cancelled credit cards will dribble through in the mail over the next month or so. I learned that, while this would have caused me no end of grousing a year ago, now I just said, "Oh, shoot." Well, actually, my language was a bit stronger than that!

Sarah had her first track meet (city level) and won her heat but did not make the finals. Her relay team ran well, too, but did not place in the end. She was really excited and I found out it is harder to watch your own kid than to do it yourself. (Some of you may recall I was a runner in another life.) Sarah's track meet, along with a piano recital, was very stressful on poor old Mummy. A couple of brother-sister teams played at the recital and I suggested to Carolyn that she could do that someday. She thought it would be nifty. Andrew, on the other hand, muttered something like, "Oh, yuck!"

Carolyn is most impressed by her big sister these days. Alan made it to the recital (a very proud daddy) and I think really enjoyed seeing Sarah do so nicely. Unfortunately, she has been having a lot of bad dreams lately, but that is what the big bed is for. My goodness, nine-year-olds have pointy knees and elbows. However, they are not nearly as much trouble in a bed as a husband.

Andrew rescued three crow babies and a mouse (well, the mouse was dead). It went like this: "Mummy, Stormy killed a crow." (Stormy is the cat next door.) I went out to see this, because cats don't normally take on crows. As it turned out, it wasn't an adult crow and it wasn't dead and it was actually three baby crows. For the next fifteen minutes, I chased baby crows into and out of the hedges and yard and field, while being dive-bombed by parent crows and while trying to evade all the young neighbourhood cats that suddenly appeared on the scene. Baby crows are not small but, thanks to Perky training, I was able to transport the critters with a tearful Andrew by my side to the local woods rather than the ground under the pine tree in our backyard. Last night, Andrew attempted to rescue a big fat mouse from Stormy, but it was DOA. This is the first time I have encountered a dead, very bloody mouse in a margarine tub in my kitchen. Andrew then buried it and I then disinfected Andrew from head to toe.

Alan and Andrew have been having a fine time lately comparing their common interest in bugs and similar creatures in the yard and at the cottage, things such as a piece of rabbit, a millipede about 8 cm long, a piece of crayfish and a chunk of bird. All this has brought about a number of neat observations about life. By Carolyn: "Mummy, when Grandma dies we can bring her home in the car and bury her in the garden?" By Andrew: "Mummy, will you and Daddy be compost someday?" Well, actually, Andrew, yes but the city prefers we put only plant matter in the compost. Very pragmatic children we have sometimes.

The symptoms of Al's disease are still there, but he is coping well for now. I sense some decrease in interest in doing stuff, but hope that a recent drop in the dose of one of the anti-seizure drugs will help. This time no food restrictions and, for those of you in the know, he'll be taking Tamoxifen (used for breast cancer as well). It should cut his estrogen levels dramatically. What that does to testosterone is not clear to me, but knowing Alan…

Moyra

Wednesday, June 16, 1999

It was a pretty hard week last week. Alan started chemo and slept a lot. Andrew went to Emergency in the middle of the night for croup. Carolyn needed antibiotics and I was pooped. On Friday, the disability insurance company sent a letter saying that it had overpaid Alan by $2,000 and could we please send it quick.

This week has been much better. Today the surgeon, for the first time, used the word *encouraging*. The radio-surgery seems to have reduced the area of enhancement. Isn't that a nice term to use for the reaction the tumour has to the dye that is injected into Al's bloodstream before the test? In other words, the tumour doesn't seem to have grown since the last scan. This is good news. It's still about 2 cm across and still pushing in the ventricle, but it didn't grow last month. We check again after another month.

Alan is doing better on the new chemo trial. He feels pretty blah but hasn't had much in the way of problems. There is some ongoing cognitive loss still, but we are working around it. Then, also today, the disability insurance company reversed its decision on the overpayment and decided that all my faxes, letters, begging and grovelling were acceptable. As a final compliment, Perky has learned the word *come*. Mind you, he only comes to me and refuses to fly to the others. Alan says this is normal in children. He has always claimed that he taught them the word *Mummy*.

Moyra

Thursday, June 25, 1999

It has been a quiet time for Alan over the last week. He has had his first cycle of the new chemo drugs and found it tiring. The nausea was well controlled by Zofran for the few days after the two intravenous treatments. Then he switched to Stemitil, which also makes him sleepy. Our house is decorated with yellow buckets strategically located, but in the end not required. The oral Tamoxifen seems to be well tolerated.

The radiation oncologist was very pleased with his handiwork from the stereotactic treatment in May, but told Alan there can be no more radiation at that particular site. This means the cancer has to recur somewhere else in order to get more radiation. The centre of the tumour was killed by the stereotactic radiation (good news), but these things grow from the surface and the surface is still active.

Moyra

Wednesday, July 7, 1999 – Alan, on MORE BOATING WITH BRAIN DAMAGE

You may remember some weeks ago I had an experience getting into our rowboat. I have since then spent a lot of time thinking about what I did wrong and how one is supposed to get into a boat. The problem was more than just untying it first. You have to keep your balance and transfer your weight smoothly from one foot to the other while stepping in. Last weekend, I tried my luck getting into the boat. Untie it first, put one leg inside while keeping your weight on the other, step in and shove off. It worked great. I had a nice row around the bay and returned to the dock. Now how to get out? Just the reverse of getting in, you say? Not so fast there. Now you are in the moving part aiming at the stationary part. My balance is not so good and my reactions are painfully slow. Somehow I turned the boat completely upside down and smacked my head on the dock on the way down ('tis but a flesh wound). Moyra has suggested I capsize the boat farther offshore where injury is less likely next time I want to get out. I'll have to give the getting-out part more thought.

Alan

Thursday, July 8, 1999

As promised, here is the update after Alan's latest CT scan, hot off the presses from 8:30 this morning. The tumour has not grown this month. That means two months of stable disease (another nice term I have learned). It's still about 2.5 cm across. It's still on the edge of the ventricle, but it's stable for now. We hope that the toxic soup of chemo that he is on is doing some good. He has been having headaches and night sweats again, and he had another very small seizure, so we had figured it was growing. The doctor says it's likely part of the chemo, since the brain swelling seems to be under control. Alan is very sleepy and can't do very much before needing to rest, but this is almost surely the result of chemo. The sleepiness worries us, since it is also the next stage of his disease.

I'm sure you all enjoyed Alan's boating story last week. Yes, he wears a life jacket all the time now, even for swimming. He is also after me to move the canoe down to the lake. I am reluctant to do so. If he can flip a stable little rowboat and whack his head on the dock in the process, what can he do in a canoe? I have been wondering whether it is possible to flip a canoe end-for-end, or will he simply do a roll over the side?

I broke my ankle last week. It is not too bad, actually, just a hairline fracture of the right fibula for which I have been allowed not to have a cast. However, I had to promise to be a good girl and not jump or play soccer or lift boats or haul on a tent trailer for at least three and up to six weeks. There goes the camping trip.

The ankle incident occurred on the day of Sarah's birthday party, when I foolishly decided to cut the grass before her party. As if eight giggling ten-year-olds would notice a messy lawn. The mower tossed out a hunk of wood about the size of a pop can split lengthwise, and my ankle turned a fascinating shade of purple within moments. The children, now expert medical types, trundled off to get ice (Andrew with Alan's help) and extra-strength Tylenol (Sarah) and a toy (Carolyn). When my ankle started to look more like a purple tennis ball on a broomstick, I capitulated and did the X-ray thing. Since I wanted a fibreglass cast (not plaster), I was band-aged and returned home. The girls were most impressed by my various purple features, including heels and, by the next day, toes, and really gave themselves their own party, since I declined to go up and down the stairs to the sleepover more than a few times. On the Monday, I was permitted to wait until Tuesday to see a specialist, who agreed that I could indeed go without a cast, since I was, by then, walking fairly well.

Alan and I must look quite a sight when we walk together into the Cancer Centre these days. Is it the lady with the gimpy foot or the guy with the fantastic scar who is off balance who is there for chemo treatment? As it turns out, Alan has held on to most of his hair so far. It has thinned quite a bit and has fallen out in the area where the big radiation beam went through last fall. He has lost all the weight gained on the high-dose Decadron regime of the fall, winter and spring, and looks pretty good. Cognitively he is doing fairly well, too. He is back to reading books in a big way, which was something he was not really able to do easily even in January and February. He finds the computer difficult to use, since his left hand is slow, but he is sending e-mail. The doctors would like to see him more active in a good way (walking, golfing – I don't think so!). We have to find a good physical activity for him. Alan figures he's walked around the block a couple of times and there is not a lot new to see. The surgeon's prescription today may be hard to fill, but I will give it serious consideration – he told me to get Alan a dog! I can hear it now: "Stupid bird, squawking all the time; damn cat, always hungry, get out of my way; shut up, dog, I'll take you out later." On that note, perhaps I will misplace that prescription.

Alan has another chemo treatment tomorrow and then another cycle in early August. We see the surgeon again on September 1. I'll send an update then unless something of interest happens in the meantime. Have a great summer and thanks, as always, for your ongoing support.

Moyra

Alan was very good at playing with children in a completely natural way. As a result, he was a big hit with all the kids at family reunions. One of his favourite summer pastimes was making dribble sandcastles. Being a child at heart, at least on the beach, and an engineer by occupation, he loved to make castles and moats and canals. He insisted that each of the children have a proper metal trowel, since plastic shovels are completely inappropriate for proper construction of beachfront fortifications. When he mastered the technique for making a dome for the castle roof, he considered it to be among his most significant lifetime achievements.

The sand at Sandbanks Provincial Park on Lake Ontario was ideal for castle building. We had often spent part of our summer vacation at Sandbanks, and this year was no exception, although we had to drive there from a cabin I rented for us. My broken ankle made our usual camping trip impossible.

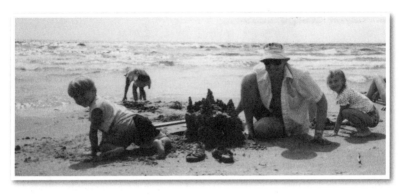

ANDREW, SARAH (AT THE WATER'S EDGE), ALAN AND CAROLYN BUILD A CASTLE
AT SANDBANKS PROVINCIAL PARK.

Wednesday, August 11, 1999

Alan is doing quite well. He sleeps a lot and is fairly grouchy (with good reason), but is doing push-ups and sit-ups in the morning these days. We had a great break at a cabin near Picton for a week in the hot weather, and then I went to Chicago to present a paper at a conference. The kids stayed with friends. Al managed, with his parents' help, on his own.

The timing was just about perfect. The day after I returned from Chicago, I drove Sarah to another friend's cottage for a weeklong visit and got back at 10:00 p.m. At 10:05, Alan had a really bad seizure. It started, we got it stopped and then it started again and was bad enough that he asked me to hold him down. I will never get used to holding him like that as his body shakes and thrashes. He remained conscious but it took another two pills before it stopped. The post-seizure paralysis lasted about 30 minutes in his left arm and he was limping the next day. Naturally, doses of his anti-seizure drug levels have now been increased.

He is still hoping and planning to present our keynote lecture in Austria in October. I am taking some time off right now, just rewriting some of the material for the paper and practising some deep breathing.

Moyra

Monday, August 30, 1999

It has been a great summer and Alan has been doing really well. He has been having weekly seizures since mid-August, likely from the chemo drugs interfering with the anti-seizure stuff.

On Saturday at the lake, I installed a plumbed vanity with a sink in the outhouse. There is still no running water, but there is a big jug of lake water for washing. I knew Alan was under the weather because he let me use all the tools. In fact, he was downright nice about it. It's always a bad sign when I can use the prized brace and bit and he merely says that he'll go read his book now. However, he perked up enough to go skinny-dipping at 11:00 p.m. and chase me around in the water. Sarah's ten-year-old visiting friend claims we are certifiable. Sunday was cool, so we had a quiet day. Alan went out in the rowboat for a long row – against my better judgment, but the guy needs something to do – and came back really beat.

On the way home he fell asleep in the car, and had a dream in which he told all of us in the car "not to slam the door as we leave." He seemed better afterwards, but at 3:00 a.m. had a massive seizure. He was in a deep sleep at the time and I still don't know whether the "Oh, shit" I heard was from a dream he was in or the realization of the problem. I stopped the seizure but it took four magic pills. He was very weak on the left, with left-side weakness and paralysis still present at 6:00 a.m. At 7:00 a.m. he had uncontrollable chills and by 8:30 his parents were here so I could take him to the hospital because by then the chills were gone and the fever was above 38°C and climbing.

So we again visited the great resort called stretcher bay for a number of hours. Alan has now been admitted to hospital. The problem is from the chemo, not the strep Sarah had last week or the infection Carolyn has this week. He has low counts of red and white blood cells and platelets. We'll have to see whether he can tolerate another cycle of this type of chemo. The upside is that the CT scan seems to show the tumour is no bigger, although the brain edema is quite a bit worse – hence, the seizures. Alan has a nice purple lip – it looks as if he has been eating blueberry pie – and bruising on his arms and is quite weak.

Moyra

Alan's disability insurance required regular submissions from his medical doctors. The word *incurable* was written on every one. The medical staff would always soften the word when they were speaking to Alan, saying things such as, "Statistics apply to the group; you are an individual" and "We want to be sure you get the financial support you need at this time." While Alan believed he would be an exception to the statistics, he also remembered overhearing a doctor telling a resident always to put things in the very best light for patients.

A typical medical statement would be like the one shown below. It reads, "If disease progression confirmed, it would be highly unlikely that Mr. Oddy would ever return to *any* form of employment. The prognosis remains poor – his disease is incurable, with short life expectancy."

A PORTION OF THE DISABILITY INSURANCE SUBMISSION IN AUGUST.

Wednesday, September 1, 1999

Alan seems to be improving quickly. His blood work today showed remarkable improvement in the white cell count. The bone marrow seems to be recovering quickly. His red cell and platelet counts are still down. The doctors hope to have him home for the weekend, although the epilepsy-type behaviour is back in his left arm, likely caused by brain swelling pushing on some electrical connection. Alan wants to get home because he has already had enough hospital food. Breakfast this morning was prunes and wilted waffles. In our 21 years of marriage, Alan has never eaten prunes!

He is on seizure watch in the hospital. This really bugs him, since it means he has to call a nurse just to use the facilities, and chemo means that when you need to go, you really need to go. I suspect he doesn't always call. He wanted me to take him for a walk today, but on seizure watch he is restricted to his room. I half expect to find him in the halls tomorrow. He is clever enough to use his short-term memory loss to his own advantage from time to time: "My room, really, you don't say. When did the doctors order that?"

Damage to his short-term memory may be caused by the swelling in the brain. He fell down on the morning of the seizure at home, but has completely forgotten it happened. (I haven't. I am the one who had to heft his body off the floor to the bed. Naturally, being Alan, he managed to wedge himself into the small space between the bedroom patio door and the bedside table when he fell. It was quite a trick getting him out of there. Fortunately, he was able to help me to some extent by using the side of his body that was not still weak from the seizure.) This means that when the nurse asked him, "Have you fallen down in the last two to three days?" Alan answered, "Nope, never fallen down," because he has no memory of it happening.

In keeping with the tradition of pet acquisition tactics when Alan isn't there to back me up (read, give me a backbone), we have acquired a mate for Perky. Sarah points out that the big S on my chest stands for Softie. Alan says it stands for Sucker. I suspect he is more correct. Pearl, a female cockatiel, joined us last night. Three sad, worried-about-Daddy children had prevailed upon me to take them to the pet store to see this bird. They have had their eyes on her for some time now. In fact, they named her almost a month ago. The name Pearl comes from the fact that she is a pearl-mutation, with lots of markings. I tell myself that the trip to the shoe store for new fall school shoes ended up costing me more than this bird did, but that only says that the children have expensive taste in shoes. In any case, Pearl is very coy and shy. For the first few hours, she huffed (bird anger) every time Perky came near. Perky was strutting around in seventh heaven. His crest was straight up and he kept showing her his beautiful wings and doing flying acrobatics. Guys are the same everywhere: see my wings; see my fast car. By today, Perky was nibbling her neck feathers and preening her tail feathers. She is still not letting him sit right next to her, but she watches him closely. At one point, he was trying to get her to join him in a bird bath. She would have none of it. She likes to have her armpits (wingpits?) rubbed, so the kids spent a lot of time early this morning stroking her underwings. If Perky figures out how to do that, she'll forgive him anything.

They shouldn't mate until the spring. (Does anyone want a cockatiel baby? One of Sarah's friends is already in line, and another one put in a pitch for a bird in the spring. I suspect they'll start working on their parents immediately. You know who you are. Be warned!) I am hoping this new bird will make things easier on Alan. Perky had become very attached to his human flock and would regularly screech and squawk to find out where the flock was (especially first thing in the morning). When I returned from Chicago, Alan had been the only flock around for several days. I guess he found it annoying to be so needed because he informed me that "The g-d bird screams in my ear and then sh...s on my shoulder. How do you want me to feel about him?" With the kids going back to school and my vacation time over, it seemed wise to get a distraction for Perky lest he end up alone with Alan near a sharp kitchen knife!

Perky spends all his time chasing Pearl around the cage. He is switching his attention from us – flightless, rather stupid and certainly ugly birds – to a winged creature from paradise with lovely yellow tail feathers. Hence, the screeching and squawking calls to find us have largely been replaced by beak gritting (bird happy sounds). Pearl has, so far, a delicate chirp and gurgles.

It looks as if Alan will be allowed to continue his chemo. Again today we were told that the tumour looked smaller. The brain edema is not so good, but should go down with an increase in his Decadron levels, which were bumped up today. This also means that his weight loss will soon be replaced by weight gain, since the Decadron is an appetite stimulant. Alan was about 190 pounds before this all started a year ago. He peaked at about 225 pounds in April, when he had the second surgery. He has been dropping since then and is now at about 180 pounds. He will see the surgeon tomorrow for a regular follow-up to assess the size of the tumour and the extent of the edema and figure out some new drug regime. Fun and games.

Moyra

Alan's sister-in-law, Yolond, was undergoing treatment for breast cancer at this time. With surgery, radiation and chemotherapy to get through, she was able to relate to Alan's situation. She and Alan chatted on the phone and exchanged e-mails from time to time when they felt up to it. I know it helped Alan to talk to someone who had some real idea of the physical and emotional issues with which he was dealing. It also gave him an outlet to vent on other matters, including his obvious frustration with me. I was under no illusions at the time about how Alan felt. I know there were times when he had simply had it with me and with all the things he was going through. I'm very grateful to Yolond for having listened so patiently.

Thursday, September 2, 1999

Alan is home again. The higher Decadron levels have given him a rush of energy, so he will drive me crazy for a while. He is already planning his weekend at the lake, and I have had to remind him that he ought to rest a bit first. He was sleeping in less than five minutes. That was our first experience of low white and red cell counts and low platelet counts. A jolly experience, to be sure. Actually, yesterday Al met a very attractive intern who asked if she could add him to her portfolio of patients. He was delighted to help out. She was very bright and, even better, she laughed at his jokes. One of the downsides of short-term memory loss is telling the same joke over and over and over.

His chemo has been delayed until next week to give his body a bit more time to recover. He is on antibiotics to prevent infection by school-aged children and wives who work at bacteria-laden universities ("Professor, I have to miss the midterm. I think I am going to throw up all over your desk.")

So our roller-coaster life continues although the dips down are not as wild as they were last year and the climbs up seem to be occurring a little more often. Alan's surgeon also now agrees that the tumour is at least no bigger, and he ventured the opinion that it might be a bit smaller. Not bad, considering that Alan was not really supposed to be with us at this point. He never did like statistics.

Moyra

Wednesday, September 22, 1999

Well, the plans for the great adventure to Europe are in place. As you know, no life is complete without doing the grand tour of Europe. We are travelling without cancellation insurance (we can't get any because Alan has a pre-existing condition). It would have cost almost $400 for cancellation insurance for the kids and me so we are living dangerously. The kids will go even if they have the flu, and we'll eat the $400 in London. Alan's nephew is staying at the house to cat- and bird-sit. Alan is really tired these days. I am very concerned that he will have trouble doing the trip, so I've stuck extra days of rest in all over the place. We are even staying over Saturday in a number of places to reduce the cost of travel (what a hardship!). Alan was miffed this morning when he realized I had his itinerary as "sleep in London" and my itinerary as "go with kids on double-decker bus, see Tower of London, have tea at Harrods, spend more money."

The kids are excited as heck. I am nervous as heck, but Alan has been living towards this conference since last September. I am thrilled he has made it this far. He is having a bit of trouble preparing the presentation. It's amazing how much is still in his head (e.g., the material gauge size used during neutron diffraction), and yet something simple like rearranging the order of three slides is exceedingly difficult for him. Even more so, I think, to have me come in and say, "Put this here, that there, rewrite this, put this there, and it's done" – poor guy.

So, a weekend of doing laundry and packing and kids as high as kites. I think we might pop down to the cabin and freeze on Saturday night.

Moyra

Monday, September 27, 1999

He made it! We are off to Europe tomorrow. I have a thesis defence to attend in Sweden and we have the paper to present in Graz, Austria. At this point, Alan is presenting it. He is doing well despite the tumour and edema. He has recovered from the low white and red cell and platelet counts that hospitalized him earlier this month. Long-term memory is still strong.

When we get back, he has another CT scan to see whether the edema is down and whether we can lower his Decadron dosages. His anti-seizure drug levels are fantastically high. The pharmacist questions them every time. For the moment, no more seizures.

Moyra

Taking a trip like this was a gamble, but Alan was doing relatively well, his doctors were supportive, and Alan wanted to present the paper. Being invited to present a keynote address at an international conference is a career milestone for researchers, and it meant a great deal to Alan, especially under the circumstances. He extracted a promise from me to get him there, no matter what.

I understood his motivation to make this trip. It was symbolic of having achieved a certain level of success and recognition, and that mattered to Alan. A colleague of ours from another university had been fighting a less aggressive form of brain cancer for over a decade. She and I talked at length several times after Alan's diagnosis. Her greatest disappointment on the professional side was not having achieved the rank of full professor before her illness resulted in long-term disability. Her deep and profound regret, despite all her other achievements, both personal and professional, impressed upon me the importance of this trip for Alan. As crazy as it was, I decided I would do my best to make it happen.

Saturday, October 2, 1999

We survived the trip over here. I am in our Swedish friends' (Lars-Erik and Eva's) kitchen talking to my computer at Carleton University. Alan slept a lot on the way over. He is confused at times about what day it is and what time it is. To my horror, he went out alone in London when he was supposed to stay in the room. He found his way back by asking directions from some workers at the back of an alley. He ignored my request that he let me do the drug stuff and took two sets of drugs at once. Other than that, he is fine.

He went with me to the Swedish Ph.D. party last night and enjoyed seeing all the old friends we made when we spent three months here in 1993 during my first sabbatical. We feel very comfortable here – like at home, everyone is very kind and helpful.

I learned more about tipping etiquette when using wheelchair service at airports. American helpers put their hand out at the end for the tip and let you know by their expression whether it is too little. In Canada, a tip is received with thanks but is not necessary. In Britain it is accepted but not looked at. In Sweden, they try to give it back.

Back to London tomorrow and then on to Austria.

Moyra

Monday, October 11, 1999: The ODDYsee

You heard from us in Luleå, Sweden, on Saturday afternoon. All was well and the one missing bag had been delivered so Carolyn had clean clothes. We always travel with a bit extra, so no big deal. At 11:00 p.m., I finished packing and went upstairs for a bit. At midnight, I checked on Alan, who told me he'd had a mild seizure. He also had a temperature of 38.2°C – we had a sick boy. Eva (a nurse) took us to the Luleå Emergency department. Alan should have had IV antibiotics, but since we had a flight in the morning to Stockholm and then London and Al was relatively strong, the doctor gave him oral antibiotics. I got him to London and put him to bed and prayed the antibiotics would work. With low white and red blood cell and platelet counts, a small cold (like we all had) is enough to flatten a chemo patient.

Next morning, Alan was sick as heck but determined to try for Austria. We tried to leave for Gatwick (via train at Victoria station) but I couldn't do it all and we missed our train. I went to the British Airways office at Victoria Station and they adopted us at customer service. I cannot say enough good things about them. They found a doctor who cleared Alan for further flight but added another whammy of antibiotics on top of what he was already taking. She, too, suggested IV and hospital, but Al was still determined to go and climbed the 36 steps to the doctor's office to prove it (and then turned off again). (Alan remembers very little of all of this, but when the very attractive doctor in Sweden said, "I'm going to look in your eyes now," he said, "Go right ahead!" and meant it. In Victoria Station, the doctor spoke mostly to me, since Alan was becoming quite weak, but Alan remarked afterward, "I wonder whether she always has those buttons undone or was it just for me?").

In any case, we were given new flights, threw our Vienna to Leibnitz train tickets in the garbage and opted for a flight to Graz, Austria (more $$$$). I'm hoping I can get a refund on the train part. British Airways even put us in business class for one flight at no extra cost so that Alan wouldn't have to walk so far back in the plane. So Alan got another of his life's wishes – to travel in an airplane with enough space to stretch out his legs.

By the time we arrived in Graz, Alan was too weak to speak much, was unable to feed himself and was paralyzed on the left so much that he couldn't hold his fingers for me to put gloves on, so he wore socks on his hands to stay warm. He was only communicating by nodding yes or no, and at one point whispered that it was a big mistake to do the trip. I was pretty much carrying him everywhere with the help of very good airline people. To get him off the flight in Vienna, I had to put my hands around his waist, and put my knees into his knees to get his legs to move. It was truly horrible and I shed a few tears in bathrooms when no one was watching.

Eventually, we made it to Leibnitz and, with the help of the conference people and our Swedish friend at the conference, we got Alan up the stairs into the magnificent old castle/convent where the conference was being held. In the middle of the night he began to improve, thank heaven. He needed to pee (warning: graphic images coming), so I hoisted him up, manhandled him to the toilet, pulled down his drawers (he tells me the worst part of all of this was the manhandling and lack of dignity, at times) and was going to help him sit when all of a sudden I was confronted by an uncontrolled fire hose of pee. I grabbed it, got it under control and was congratulating myself on my ability to work one of those things when I realized that the "Oh, shit" he had said was not from the early use of the high-pressure hose but a more literal problem. The beautiful doctor in

London had warned me – so we added Imodium (an over-the-counter anti-diarrhea medication) to his list of new drugs.

Alan was beginning to recover and thought he could watch me give the presentation, but a new problem appeared. None of our bags had made it to the conference and he was running out of anti-convulsant medication. I had an extra day's worth of drugs on hand, but with all the confusion when he became ill I'd forgotten to switch over to box two for week two, and we were now on our last dose. All the Austrian staff were marvellous. With the help of the hard copy of the prescription (carried from Canada just in case), we were able to get his drugs in Austrian form, but not until after the presentation. Alan became very nervous about having a seizure while I was talking, so he took a sublingual Ativan. This meant he got very sleepy, so he asked for help and our new and old friends took him back to the room (where another new friend was watching the children) and I gave the talk – wearing my travel clothes, not my super confidence-building power suit. I gave the talk pretty cold, not having had a chance to look it over, but at least having spent a fair amount of time helping Alan to prepare it. It was very well received. At that point, I was numb. Who needed a power suit? I had just carried my husband across Europe.

Alan had the strength to go to the conference dinner that night in a wheel-chair and to lunch the next day. Sarah was put in charge of her siblings, since I felt it was safe to leave them with her in the room just down the hall. She earned lots of babysitting money and was happy counting her new wealth. At the lunch, the kids stayed for a while and then popped in and out a few times to check on me. Later, Sarah even stayed with her dad just to watch him. It was a heavy load to put on her, but she seemed to grow taller for the responsibility. I hope it will be a long time before we need her to be sixteen again (perhaps when she is sixteen!). So, at least Alan saw the people to see and made it to the conference. He is disappointed he didn't do the talk, though. Even though we have been partners in research for nearly ten years, there is still some competition between us, and that was to be his address, not mine.

By the time we arrived in London on Thursday, Alan was able to walk on his own a little. He could climb a few stairs and get around our room, but he didn't come on any of our sightseeing. He did, however, come out for dinner with our friends from Cambridge, as we had arranged before the trip.

The kids, especially Sarah, were tremendous. It is quite something to see your ten-year-old holding her daddy's hand and helping him to find a spoon to use or helping him to a seat since he doesn't know the way. She also babysat for me and, more than once, took Andrew and Carolyn to the bathroom. I had to rely on her in places like Gatwick, Heathrow and other large dangerous areas. Normally I wouldn't have done it, but she is a bright little thing and acted very responsibly. At another point, as Alan recovered a bit, he would have trouble opening something. Carolyn would say, "That's okay, Daddy, I can do it for you," and she did.

Andrew also did his bit and on several occasions stayed with Alan alone, when Alan wasn't much of an adult, except in size. He agreed to stay with Daddy and watch the bags (as one must do in Europe). The kids amazed me with their strength and coping abilities, including being patient for five hours in Victoria Station while I tried to sort things out.

So, here we are back in Canada but in the wrong time zone again. Andrew appeared in the bedroom at 4:00 a.m. Ottawa time (9:00 a.m. London time). It will be a long time before we do a trip like that again. While Alan is on chemo he is likely to have these episodes. What it means for more chemo is unclear. The doctors had said that he couldn't have too many more bad spells, since it indicates he is not tolerating the chemo well.

Moyra

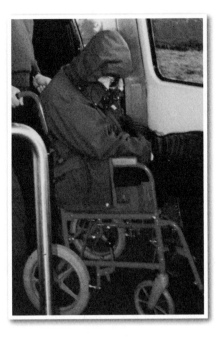

ALAN ALL BUNDLED UP AND IN A WHEELCHAIR, PUSHED BY A BRITISH AIRWAYS ATTENDANT.

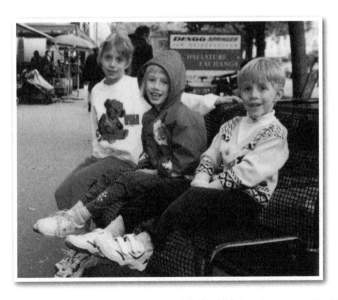

SARAH, CAROLYN AND ANDREW TAKE A BREAK WHILE OUT FOR A WALK IN LEIBNITZ, AUSTRIA.

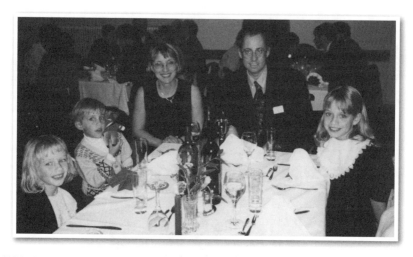

CAROLYN, ANDREW, MOYRA, ALAN AND SARAH AT A FANCY CONFERENCE DINNER IN AUSTRIA.

I knew before we left that taking this trip was a gamble. Indeed, I remember it as a kind of hell-ride. Even so, the decency and compassion of the people we encountered – the airline agents, our Swedish friends, the doctors, the pharmacist and the staff at the conference – made the trip precious in its own right.

The conference venue was a castle and former bishop's residence. While there were modern hotel rooms, we stayed in the old convent portion of the residence, which could accommodate family groups. If there are earthly angels, the sister who cared for our rooms surely must have been one, because without a word of English, she let me know that I could count on her for help. Years later, we still exchange Christmas cards – she in German and I in English.

Despite all the difficulties, the trip was worth every moment. The children remember things like playing in the park in Sweden, running down the hill at the castle, watching the Queen's horse guard in London and being bumped up to business class, just as much as they remember all the problems of their dad being sick. There is something to this idea of building memories.

Tuesday, October 12, 1999 – Alan to a friend who attended the conference in Austria

I'm very proud of Moyra and even more deeply in her debt than before. I had the easy part – just look sick and flop from one wheelchair to the next.

Alan

Tuesday, October 12, 1999

Well, the good news is that the tumour has not grown again, which makes almost four months. The edema is under control, so some of the drug doses can come down a bit. Alan's platelet count is still too low to allow the next cycle of chemo, since there is a small risk he will bleed into the tumour. So we have another week's delay before continuing.

The medical oncologist seems most pleased with himself. Every time he sees one of these CT scans he just about grows taller in front of us. He is delighted that someone is doing well on this experimental trial, I think. Perhaps he has others doing well, too. I must ask him.

After a good night's sleep I feel much more ready to take on the world again, but I think we'll postpone any travel for a good long time.

Moyra

Wednesday, October 20, 1999

Alan has not recovered enough from the previous cycle of chemo to have more. His platelet counts especially are way too low, almost at the level of needing a blood transfusion. However, the break seems to have improved his appetite a bit, at least. So he may gain back a few pounds. He is getting down to his wedding weight (I never left it, of course) and is skin and bones to me.

Al, Sarah and I have had our flu shots. Since Al's white blood cell count is so low he is at risk from all kinds of infection, even Andrew and Carolyn will get a pediatric dose of the flu shot next week.

Moyra

Monday, November 15, 1999

On my way home from seeing Andrew (yes, Andrew) in hospital last night, I looked up at the sky and said, "I'm just about at my limit." Then I had a good chat with my favourite tree in the woods between the house and the hospital.

Alan is fine, thank heaven, because Andrew is not. It's a good thing Alan is in the good two weeks of the month. I forbade him yesterday to do one of his immune system crash-things or to have any seizures.

Andrew has a serious infection called ocular cellulitis. It has a few nasty bits in common with the flesh-eating strep but is not a strep infection. The school called on Friday because he had a headache. A few hours later I took him to Emergency (he was spiking a fever). I reassured myself that the long wait meant he was not that sick and, in fact, after tests, we were sent home, after being told he had a virus but to come back if it worsened. At 3:00 p.m. on Saturday Andrew refused to open his eyes (and only willingly reopened the good eye today). That's when I knew the level of pain involved.

That night, the children's Emergency section had every kid and their dog in there. There were two infant resuscitations, a bunch of broken teen-age bones from a girls' hockey game, and kids holding buckets in every corner. So from 6:00 p.m. to nearly midnight we waited while Andrew's eye puffed up and up and up.

Finally, we saw a very conservative doctor who treated me like the stu-pidest mother in the world. The doctor told me it was meningitis and that a spinal tap had been ordered. I declined that procedure until a second opinion could be found, since Andrew had no stiffness in his neck at all. The second opinion said it wasn't meningitis, but was maybe a bad virus. I said, "How about bloodwork to see if he is cooking something?" Boy, did Andrew ever not approve of being threaded (the term the nurses use for getting an IV line in). Then things really got rolling.

The blood test results came back in about 30 minutes and showed a big infection. Andrew started IV antibiotics and he had a CT scan that scared him into complete co-operation. He is five going on ten, and he put together this complex idea: Daddy, headache, fell down, emergency room, CT scan, brain cancer, big sickness.

Sunday morning brought ophthalmology, more waiting, and the eye test from hell. It's really hard to tell whether a kid has good vision at the best of times, but Andrew refused to open his sore eye. I could hardly blame him, but I pried his eye open and he looked at the pictures. After that he told me he was "never going to open that eye again, ever."

Sarah, Carolyn and Alan hung out at home here (thank you, God, for neighbours and friends). Sarah, my accounting genius, knows exactly how much babysitting money she is owed. I pulled some social-worker types out of their Sunday chairs and demanded help so I could get home to take care of things there (make sure Alan was up on his anti-convulsant levels), and it worked. The hospital provided (and is right now providing) a sitter just to keep Andrew company in his room. I know I guessed right because Andrew said later that he didn't want to be left alone in a hospital (the Daddy-factor, I suppose).

Andrew is much better today. We are still talking possible blindness but the ophthalmologist seems to feel it is much less likely than did the emergency doctor. However, Andrew got up to walk around today with me, on his own legs, and started to play with a toy, and shouted at me when I went out of the room without telling him. So I think we have crossed into safer territory.

I have asked again about having a hospital pass to allow Andrew to come and go for the IV treatments so I could at least keep an eye on the family a bit more. The nurses (love those nurses) seem to think it is done often enough that it can be made to work, especially since we live so close.

So, we have five days at least of intravenous antibiotics and the usual number of follow-up tests to check Andrew's sight. Thank goodness I am on sabbatical this year. In the room last night with Andrew, I was reading a Ph.D. thesis for a defence I had agreed to sit on in December – it's amazing how a good read like that can actually help one achieve sleep in a chaotic environment.

So, I'll tuck Alan in for his nap and head back to the hospital. Alan has been troubled by some of his recent cognitive losses. He forgot how to tie his shoes the other day but did manage to relearn it the same day. He really objects to being stupid. Of course, he is not stupid, but I guess that is the way it feels. He occasionally blurts out something not very helpful, such as "I can't even do what you can do." I try to take it in the nicest way.

Alan has always been an interesting guy. He figured his own work wasn't all that great, but it was a heck of a lot better than anyone else's.

Chemo cycle 6, the last of this trial, begins in less than two weeks. He had a lot of trouble getting through cycle 5; he felt wretched and had some vision problems, such as double vision. One day he called me at work to tell me the pictures were sliding down the walls.

Moyra

Thursday, November 18, 1999

Well another week has passed in the never boring life of this family. Andrew and I were granted a pass to come and go from his hospital room for his IV treatments. Andrew has exceeded expectations and did not develop any of the threatened dire consequences: he can see and the double vision is receding slowly (only two televisions when he looks left). His eyelid is droopy, but that is because he did the equivalent of carrying twins with his eyelid. The infection did not spread to the brain. The doctors delightedly let him go home provided the new oral drugs stay down. If not, it's back to the IV.

He was released from hospital late today but will be on powerful antibiotics for another couple of weeks to prevent a regrowth of the bacteria that did this. As yet, we still don't know what bug it was.

So tonight I will not sleep with the father of another child. Somehow I thought it would be more romantic than it was. In case you think I'm serious, he was in the chair on the other side of the room. His kid is having complications from a kidney transplant.

Moyra

Thursday, December 2, 1999

Alan has had his last IV chemo treatment of this clinical trial. The last of the six 4-week cycles and various delays is now coming to an end. This cycle has been quite good in terms of Alan tolerating things. His fatigue level has been much better and he has been able to putter in the workshop a bit more. On the downside, he has been depressed at the length of the treatment. It has been steady now for over a year and it's hard to keep one's spirits up, especially when things are harder to do and understand and one gets muddled about what day it is. Also, I guess it really bugs a guy to watch his wife have fun installing a new light fixture and putting up Christmas lights. The seizures have not gone away but appear to be milder and have fewer side effects than before. He had one at home on his own earlier this week but was able to handle it.

In other news, we bought a piano! It's a 1945 Willis, a beautiful piece of Canadiana that sounds wonderful even when playing children's music. It turns out I did not forget everything my mother taught me and I can still play a bit (in fact, better than Sarah for the moment). It took some furniture rearranging but the piano now dominates the living room. Sarah loves it, so it has become part of the family therapy.

The church next door has made contact and Sarah has joined their Christmas choir. Pastor Frank pops over every now and again to chat with Alan. They have great discussions on souls, God, etc. Alan is not sure how to react to the interest in his soul but figures it can't do any harm.

Andrew is well. The hospital gave him the all-clear last week. There is no permanent damage to his eye and he longer sees two of me when he looks sideways. The hospital sees several cases of ocular cellulitis each year, so it was well understood, but it still took a while to diagnose, as you know. I sure was happy to see the second IV drug change the course of the infection when the first did not seem to be working.

Alan has a CT scan on December 16. We'll know the results just before Christmas. The oncologist is not suggesting anything in particular at this point. Alan has had just about everything he can: he had the first surgery, standard radiation, boost radiation, two 6-week cycles of standard chemo, second surgery, stereotactic radiation and six 4-week cycles of an experimental clinical trial. Normally, what comes next is the wait-and-see phase, but we are asking for more treatment. Perhaps not this chemo, but at least an angiogenisus inhibitor (stops blood-vessel growth). Alan is on Tamoxifen at the moment (at a higher dose than for breast cancer) but it ends in a few days.

Moyra

Monday, December 13, 1999 – to friends who gave us the gift of snow-blowing service

Merry Christmas to you all and thank you for your very generous Christmas present. I haven't quite figured out how to spend it just yet and I'll try to explain why. I'm sure the mechies with an aero bent will understand my dilemma. For the last ten years, since children came on the scene, Alan has hogged the snow blower and all the fun of pushing around a big noisy machine and getting gas on one's fingers in the cold. "That's okay, dear, you take care of the little ones and I'll go out in the cold and do the terrible deed." For us mechies, there is a natural genetic flaw that means we actually get a real thrill out of driving one of those babies. Not to mention (for me in particular) the small satisfaction of watching Alan give the kids breakfast while I roll around the driveway in a glory of moving, swirling snow.

On the other hand, there are times when a driveway full of snow is just a bit more load than I can take on – say, when Alan is having an immune-system crash and someone has promised I will bake four dozen cookies for the special thing at school.

If you all agree, what I propose is that I will hire the local guy(s) to do perhaps Tuesday and Friday snowstorms (I teach those days – I decided to teach a course this year so I'll have one less to teach next year) or clean out the end of the driveway after the plow goes by – that is one thing that really drives me buggy. Once I've sorted out the details I'll let you know.

We really appreciate your care and concern.

Moyra

Tuesday, December 21, 1999

Usually one refers to a newborn baby as "a little miracle," but today Alan's doctor referred to Alan's tumour – more specifically, the lack of growth – as a miracle. Once again it is stable and, although it is still 1.5 cm across and 2 cm long, it has not grown now since about June! As the oncologist said, "A couple more like you and I'll write a paper!" He was indeed very pleased with himself. So, here we are, sixteen months from diagnosis and half a year past the day Alan wasn't supposed to be with us anymore. Not bad, eh? (As we Canadians say.)

Alan was given several choices of what to do next: do nothing and wait, take high-dose Tamoxifen, or try a low-dose ongoing chemo (Temodal). Since his blood counts are still the pits from the last chemo, he opted for the Tamoxifen and now takes another ten pills a day. It's made for breast cancer therapy at about 20 mg/day, so to get the high dose he needs ten pills. The pharmacist was alarmed by the number of tablets he had to get for Alan. In fact, we exhausted the pharmacy's supplies. The newest ten will be downed with the other fifteen Alan already ingests each day. There will be some lousy side effects – hot flashes, for instance (that'll be fun to watch, there is sort of a neat justice there, watching a guy go through menopause, nausea and other such things), but no more bone marrow damage as the chemos have caused. We've been told that the first chemo (January to March 1999) did permanent damage to Alan's bone marrow. The experimental trial has done only temporary damage, as is shown by his low levels of platelets and red and white cells. His lips look really pale these days. I have suggested he try a bit of lipstick and blush but I got a really dirty look for that. Gals getting chemo can have special makeup lessons called something like "look good, feel better," but I guess few guys take advantage of the skills taught there.

On the emotional side, Alan has just about had it with being sick, and it's showing in many ways. The other day he sat down in the bed and said, "I'm fed up with the cat. I'm fed up with the children and I'm fed up with…." He stopped there, but it was clear I was next on the list. At least he was able to stop before it came out. I hope that as the effects of the chemo trial fade, he'll have more strength both physically and emotionally. I know that I am also weary of it all. Some days it takes a lot of strength to paste the smile back on my face long enough for it to take. Alan asked this morning (I was just a tad grumpy) whether I hadn't slept well last night. Of course, I wake up at every burp, toot and whistle from him, so a good night's sleep is a rarity at the best of times. If his burps, toots and whistles are too loud, I am joined in the bed by three children, who also don't sleep well at times. When Alan snores (not often now after the surgery last summer to reduce his vibrating throat), both Andrew and Carolyn turn up with bad dreams, as happened last night. Perhaps with this latest low toxicity therapy we will all get a bit of a breather from the intensity of continual doctors' appointments and treatment.

Several of you have asked about the birds. Alan refers to them as a "bloody nuisance," so you can guess that he does not respond well when the doctor suggests (as he did again today) that Alan get a dog to give him a reason to go for a walk. There is even a member of the family who has a spare dog but Alan is fairly strong on this: "NO BLOODY WAY!" Alan figures he suffers enough with the current regime of one cat, two birds, five fish and four other roommates. In the morning the ritual from Alan sounds a bit like this: "Jeez, stupid cat, shut up and I'll feed you. Okay, okay, you damn birds; you shut up, too, and I'll feed you, too."

Perky has developed an interest in buzzing Sandy, the elderly cat. Several times I have watched this suicidal bird fly in low and fast over the sleeping cat, which inevitably wakes up and slowly raises an eye or a paw. The bird's wingbeats are strong enough to put out a candle (that is another story) and move loose papers, so he wakes up the cat. Every now and again, Sandy takes an active interest in the antics of this silly bird and sits up to watch the flight path more closely. You can almost see the precise mathematical calculations being processed by the old cat brain. He may be old but he's not dead yet. Pearl, the female bird, is slowly regrowing her flight feathers from her clipping last summer at the pet store. She can now fall slowly to the floor while making slight forward progress. She has taken to leaping off the cage or the perch and going for a walkabout through the house. Alan found her halfway down the basement stairs a few days ago and I found her walking along the bedroom floor with the not-dead-yet cat stalking her from the bed above. I rescued the silly bird and distracted the cat.

Sarah has developed quite a love of the piano and will now avoid homework, except for math (which she prefers), by practising. I think the electronic keyboard may have had its day, since even the two little guys hardly touch it now. All three kids are waiting for Santa and are fit to be tied each night at bedtime.

So, we wish you a happy, healthy (especially) Christmas and New Year. Alan's next CT scan is in February, so there should be more news then. Thank you for your support over the last year plus a bit. I couldn't have done it without you.

Moyra

Our Christmas present this year was a stable tumour. It was a far better Christmas than our first Christmas with cancer, but still stressful, since, again, we were told more than once to prepare for it to be our last together. I decided that a better approach was to go with the flow. I made less of an effort to make special memories and more of an effort to simply enjoy what we had.

4

January to August 2000
STABILITY

My sense of the door closing lessened during this time, when Alan's tumour was stable. Stable disease, as the doctors call it, is a period of time when there is little change. Nothing gets better but nothing gets worse, either. In our case, it gave us a bit of time to regroup, gather our strength and try to enjoy what we still had. Rather than stable disease, Alan and I preferred the engineering term unstable equilibrium. We knew that things could go completely off the rails at any time.

The most difficult part continued to be dealing with Alan's anger. Because he felt reasonably well, he expected everything to be as it once had been. He did not like all the limitations he encountered. His physical limitations were becoming extremely frustrating and emotionally he could not understand why his children were withdrawing from him. He wanted so much to be a father that he often forgot to be a daddy. Once again, I found some help for Sarah and managed to convince Alan to let me do the day-to-day child rearing. However, all of this, combined with my reminders to Alan to use his left arm or to take his pills, and any number of other things, did not do much for our relationship. Fortunately, he agreed to see a psychotherapist and that gave him a much-needed outlet.

For my part, being a research geek became more and more important as Alan's treatment became less medically standard. I was there to see the day-to-day effects of his medications and their interactions. As a result, I was often the person who chased related medical research and initiated (with his doctor's approval, of course) changes in his medications.

Wednesday, January 19, 2000

Alan has had a difficult month emotionally. I think, having ended chemo, he sort of expected that things would be better, but he started right into the Tamoxifen and the side effects are a nuisance.

The first two weeks were okay, but by week three he had bad neurotoxicity, manifested by double vision and dizziness. I was able to control the double vision by reducing one of his anti-convulsants (the double vision occurred on the days with the higher of an alternating dose) but couldn't get rid of the dizziness. The folks in the Cancer Centre triage office suggested it was disease progression, since they had never heard of dizziness being a side effect.

I had a library search done and, sure enough, up popped dizziness as a big problem in high dose Tamoxifen, particularly for people also taking the anti-seizure medication Dilantin, as Alan does. By then, of course, Alan had fallen into the bathtub (from standing beside it). As he pondered how to get out he was grateful for (and cursing at the same time) the cleverness of his wife, who had insisted that the occupational therapist put an arm-support-rail-thingy in the bathtub. With his doctor's agreement, I pulled him off the Tamoxifen for 24 hours and then, once he wasn't dizzy, started ramping it up again. We have to get to at least 160 mg/day (eight pills) to be in the therapeutic range. He is stuck at 120 mg now for a couple of days. I'll try 140 mg tomorrow. My favourite quote from all this was a medical oncologist asking *me* whether I knew or had read of dizziness being a side effect. In any case, it has all made Alan pretty pissed off at the world – a reasonable reaction, but a tad tricky to live with. Since February has always been a hard month for him (February blahs), I am not all that keen on getting to February.

The occupational therapist is going to help Alan try to regain natural use of his left arm so that he doesn't leave it hanging around all the time. She tells me I am supposed to cue him every time I see him not using it properly. I said I would try but that he might just bite my head off. I gather it is typical for husbands to hate their wives giving them constant direction. I will have to ride this teeter-totter very carefully.

The kids have responded to Al's emotional behaviour as you might expect – by turning more and more to me and less and less to Alan. I woke up this morning with three kids crammed into my part of the bed. Naturally, this sort of withdrawal makes Alan even more upset. Fortunately, there is usually one of the children who feels a bit closer to him for a while. In December it was Andrew who would sit with Daddy, until Alan took away Andrew's allowance for two weeks. Andrew, who didn't even know what he had done wrong, reacted as you might expect and now won't go anywhere with Alan, lest he lose more allowance. Carolyn stayed away in December but is closer to Alan now and is giving him lots of kisses. Sarah, bless her heart, is just trying to keep from catching the grumbles that seem pretty constant. I think she is coping well but I've given her lots of activities this term to help redirect her from Alan's illness.

So, what's next? Alan will stay on Tamoxifen until we see his doctor on January 31. If he can't tolerate it, we'll have to try something else. The CT scan is in early February. By the way, now that chemo is over, the Decadron, which keeps the swelling down, is kicking back in as an appetite stimulant. Alan is eating like a horse again. His weight is coming back up fast (from a low of 160 pounds). He should fit his clothes again soon, but before long they'll be too tight.

Moyra

Wednesday, January 26, 2000 – Alan on dizziness and anger

This is just a quick news flash. Not a hot flash; those are very different. I am currently taking Tamoxifen in huge doses as an angiogenesis inhibitor to prevent growth of new blood vessels. It is also an estrogen suppressor, not that I've ever had to worry about that. It is the standard treatment for breast cancer and many women taking it report menopause-like side effects, such as hot flashes. Being difficult and never following the pack, I have my own side effects. It makes me incredibly dizzy, with double vision so bad I can't pick up a mug of coffee, much less read. Yesterday I pitched myself head first into the bathtub, landing on my shoulder luckily (maybe not so lucky, as long as it looks accidental). Fortunately, the occupational therapist had installed a bath rail the day before or I'd still be there! It's amazing how easy it is to get stuck in odd places when your arms and legs aren't 100 percent functional.

Alan

I'm sorry if I was too surly today when you called. We are back to adjusting drug dosages again and my Dilantin levels are too high. It makes my temper much worse than normal. I also nearly tore off a key in a jammed door lock today. I stopped with the tear halfway across. Just in time!

Alan

Thursday, February 3, 2000 – Alan on anger, to his close friend Peter

Moyra says I shouldn't have snapped your head off the last time you called. The truth is you're just about the last friend I've got left. I've been in such a foul mood for some weeks now that it's a wonder my head is still attached. Unfortunately, when I think of the number of people I despise who will out-live me, out-earn me, see more places and do more fun things, my blood begins to boil. Everybody here urges me to be thankful for what I have. That's like the guy who always said, "It could be worse," meaning, it could be happening to me instead of you. I know you have to play the hand you are dealt, but it seems like fate's been dealing from the bottom of the deck in my case for the last 20 years.

Alan

Friday, February 4, 2000 – Alan on anger

Got your voice mail. Thanks. It's been a rough month for all of us. The doctors tell me there are typically six stages to a terminal illness: denial, anger, acceptance, bargaining and two more I can't recall (one is probably being dead). There has been a lot of anger and tension here, as you might expect. Sarah is having a very hard time of it. Being the eldest child, much is expected of her. The psychotherapist I am seeing says that Moyra will be going through the same six stages, which accounts for the sparks when we are both angry at the same time. The psychotherapist also says that there are three things that have a bearing on survival. First, the victim must have a good support network of friends and family. Next, the victim must have a sense of humour and, finally, needs to believe in some higher power. Two out of three is not bad, but it wouldn't get me into graduate school.

Alan

Actually, there are five stages in a terminal illness; I was told that some or all could occur in any order or in any combination. They are denial and isolation; anger; bargaining; depression and helplessness; and acceptance. None of these really covers the fighting-for-your-life phase or the fighting-for-your-husband's-life phase. Maybe that is what Alan meant by the sixth stage.

Sunday, February 6, 2000

Several of you have asked about the results of the CT scan that we should have received by now. Well, the oncologist is in the sunny south, so Al's appointment was moved to February 15. We will have more information then.

Alan is still struggling with, in his words, a foul mood. It worries me because his mood was quite bad last year as the tumour grew and grew. He is likely also in the anger phase of dealing with his cancer. It's understandable, of course, but very difficult to live with at times. Sarah is especially fragile right now. We're hoping a March break with friends will help her decompress for a few days. We all sure need a holiday, but you can't escape this thing. It goes everywhere with you. A friend described it as a bit like a giant farting gorilla that is in the room making stinks while everyone is pretending it's not there.

Alan is getting a few morning headaches, also a bad sign. On the upside, he has done a full push-up for the first time in about a year. (He hates doing what used to be called girls' push-ups.) He is now tolerating the minimum therapeutic dose of Tamoxifen. I doubt we'll try to get to 200 mg/day; 160 mg seems to be the limit. He is dizzy sometimes, off balance sometimes, but otherwise not too bad. He is doing tai chi which, while challenging, seems to be helping quite a bit with his balance and is an excuse to go do something. He actually gets out several times a week to do neat stuff – a movie, or a museum, or for coffee.

Alan is in pretty unusual territory. He is doing much better than expected and is now out of the range of standard treatments. We are flying by the seat of our pants and contributing to the science of cancer treatment.

Moyra

Monday, February 7, 2000

Sarah is seeing a psychologist again. It seems to help. She saw her last year every two weeks after Alan was diagnosed, but stopped over the summer (at her own request). I called the school just after Christmas and re-established contact when I sensed she was at her limit again. She's doing a little extra testing to determine the level of anxiety and risk of depression. I told the psychologist that Sarah's level of anxiety will be the same as any kid whose family is in difficulty – divorce, separation, illness, moving to a new city. My goal is for Sarah to come out of this as best she can. The social worker talks about "inflicting no harm."

I also told Alan to lay off the discipline and leave it to me but, as you know, that is very hard for a hubby to do. Unfortunately, the grump comes out before the thoughtful words do. He can't help it, I know, but it can be hard on us all. The last few days have been a bit better than last week. I had to bite hard on my own tongue when Alan turned around at one point and told me to screw off. That was a first in this marriage. I think he must have known that he had gone too far, because he was much more easygoing the next day.

The little guys seem to be pretty good for now, but no doubt they'll need help at some point, especially Andrew. It can't be good for a little fellow to have as his role model an almost always angry man. I will have to try to get Andrew some good guy gymnastic teachers and swim instructors, I think. I hope Alan will pass through this stage and into something gentler soon.

Moyra

Dr. L., our family doctor, was in the process of converting her family medical practice to a practice in psychotherapy. It was good timing for us, since she had been helping Alan deal with his depression for several years and agreed to stay with us, in particular with Alan, for the duration of his illness. Alan's oncologist recommended that Alan see a psychiatrist, but Alan refused, saying that I was the one with the psychiatric problems!

I suppose in some respects he was correct. I was going through the gamut of emotions: anger, fear, helplessness and utter frustration with a situation that was unlikely to improve, ever. I was fortunate to have a number of close friends and family members to talk to, and I also found a new family doctor to help me. Alan and I were on different roads, and we needed different kinds of help.

Monday, February 7, 2000

Alan is seeing a psychotherapist whom we both respect. His oncologist suggested a psychiatrist, but Alan refused that idea outright, so he does the therapy thing every two weeks. I can't see that it does any good, but at least he has someone other than me to talk to.

I expect the drugs are part of the problem. I know that his personality has changed due to the ice cream scoop (his words) in his head. I fully understand the anger at his situation. I can't even begin to imagine what he has to get through each day. I have enough stress just waking up each morning, knowing it will be with us again today. I know we are on different paths; we have to be. He needs to work on himself. I have to hold everything else in place.

Moyra

Monday, February 7, 2000 – Alan to his cousin Janet, who also had a brain tumour, on depression

People really should talk more. I suffered with depression for years before getting any help because I was too stubborn. I am certain it wrecked my career and nearly finished my marriage. (Perhaps that's where Moyra gets her strength; she's already seen the worst.) I well remember sitting at my desk during my post-doc weeping! These problems are supposed to run in families, especially those of above average intelligence! I still hear people tell me that I shouldn't rely on drugs but get a strong grip on myself. Not only did I try it for years without success, but also no one would say the same thing to a diabetic. We both have chemical deficiencies that require medication!

Alan

Monday, February 14, 2000

Alan had a pretty bad seizure in the middle of the night (3:00 a.m.). He didn't even wake up for this one until, of course, he realized I was shoving drugs into his mouth. The left side paralysis is easing now (3:00 p.m.) and he is able to walk on his own. His memory of the last twelve hours is toast, but he seems to be filling in the gaps now. The seizure prevented any Valentine's Day celebrations. (Alan is not a fan of Valentine's Day, so this is a good thing.)

I am hoping that it is just that his anti-convulsant levels were too low. We lowered them because of the Tamoxifen. I'll get the blood work back tomorrow and will know better then. He has been enjoying getting out with friends and family the last few weeks. This is going to be an emotional setback for him. He went out with the boys on Friday night and he really enjoyed talking to them over a no-buzz beer.

I'm feeling pretty low over this. No doubt I'm just tired from his illness and the fact that my research program is struggling right now as I try to merge two massive pieces of work – two years of Al's with two years of mine – and move forward. It is not going well right now and I want to chuck the entire career in the trash (can't do that, though; I need the money). I have been expecting seizures to start but I live always in hope that he will live to see his children grow up a bit more. It's exhausting, always living on the edge like this.

Moyra

Tuesday, February 15, 2000

The news is good. Again, the tumour has not grown. It isn't any smaller, but it has not grown. The doctor is just tickled pink again and quite delighted with the technical paper he is cooking up for some conference somewhere. We had a nice discussion about drug levels, dizziness and double vision, and I was the one who suggested what changes should be made to the various doses. What a strange position to be in.

His mood is still grumpy but perhaps this news will help. Typically, he is very unpredictable in the post-seizure stage and is likely to turn on a power tool, say the radial arm remover, because he wants to. Naturally, with his memory still impaired, he forgets things such as falling flat on his face just 30 minutes earlier because his balance was bad and his left arm was not working. Of course, in the post-seizure phase he is also likely to tell me to go to hell when I remind him that he ought not to use power tools for at least a week. Actually the doctors don't want him using them at all, but that is a lost cause. I don't even try to control that, but I think he ought to be past the falling-down stage at a minimum. He had about six falls yesterday. This does not contribute to either of us being in a good mood.

Alan's nemises, the two birds, are in fine form lately chirping up a great noise the moment the sun appears in the front window. Perky has extended his cat-baiting experiments to biting (yes, biting) the cat's neck just for fun. The poor old cat missed getting the feathers but the bird had a mouthful of cat fur! Alan, against his better judgment, has rescued this silly bird from the floor while the old-but-not-dead cat follows behind, waiting for the right moment. Pearl is more of a homebody and does a marvellous imitation of a crow when she is trying to summon the male. Often this crow screech is timed to drive Alan to distraction, say, while he is trying, with shaking hands, to bring a spoon laden with scalding soup to his mouth.

The kiddies are doing well through this stage for the moment, although we worry about Sarah, who is pretty much exhausted from trying to keep from pissing off her dad and being good and not fighting with her siblings. I can sure appreciate her position, because it is exhausting living with this thing on a daily basis. I think I am doing pretty well and then I realize that I am constantly living on the edge, waking up to give Alan drugs, for example, making decisions on the fly as the seizure progresses.

However, the tumour has not grown, so we are not losing the war yet. The category of his illness is still incurable/terminal. I still shudder when I see those words on his paperwork. But each day puts him in a different statistical pile, an outlier, in fact, and that is good. Alan has always been a bit of an outlier.

Next CT scan is in late March.

Moyra

Saturday, March 4, 2000

This happened to Andrew last summer. He put his own shoes on, on the wrong feet, his own sweatpants with his underwear on the outside, à la Batman, and a muscle shirt, back to front. He and Moyra went to the grocery store. They were standing in the checkout line and the lady behind them said, "I've had days just like that myself."

Alan

Monday, March 6, 2000 – Alan, with a high school confession to Tom

I have something to confess after all these years. It's not a bad thing I want to admit to, but rather it was probably my greatest coup! I have had to keep silent all these years, for obvious reasons, and can't do it anymore. Do you remember Clive in our class? In grade 11, on the first day of a mixed Health class, the teacher sent a sheet of paper around so we all could write our names down. There may even have been a seating plan; I don't recall. When it got around to me I noticed that Clive and I were using the same ballpoint pen so I closed off his "C" and it became an "O." The teacher read out the names and got to "Olive." whereupon the whole class nearly died laughing. The teacher wanted to know who had doctored the name list, but whoever did it knew their life wasn't worth spit, so no one, until now, did.

Alan

Tuesday, March 21, 2000 – Alan on faith and God

God may be good, but she has a malicious sense of humour. After I completed my Ph.D. I had a lot of trouble getting a job. I was basically backed into starting my own consulting business for lack of anything else. On the night of our 20th wedding anniversary, I told Moyra that I was happy, that things had actually worked out for the best. I wouldn't have enjoyed being a professor, and working for a government research lab requires developing a taste for shit that I never mastered. Anyway, next morning when I started to shave I had my first seizure. Who says God doesn't listen? She just doesn't always give you what you want!

Alan

Alan actually had better luck job hunting than this comment about a cheeky female God suggests. He really meant fate here, and fate did not offer the career choices he particularly wished to have, when he wished to have them. We knew that we could end up in places we never expected to be. We had already experienced career changes due to outside circumstances, since a recession and potential layoffs were responsible for our decision to take our doctorates. When we graduated, there were fewer career choices available than we had hoped. Our desire to remain close to family, at a time when my dad's Alzheimer's was becoming severe, limited even those. Later, as my university career stabilized and we had children, the idea of uprooting everyone and everything would have required a special opportunity. As logical as all of that was, it still bothered Alan.

Tuesday, March 28, 2000

It has been a long wait for this latest CT scan and its results but the results are good. Once again, there has been no growth. There is some edema (cause unknown) that likely accounts for the cognitive losses I've seen this month, and perhaps the headaches, too. So, we move up to an MRI next month to see what is going on at a more detailed level. The CT scan shows some calcification of the tumour and that is good news.

The words *remission* and *cure* have not been mentioned yet. But it's good news again. To be honest, with the three seizures in the last month I was wondering. One seizure was caused by a missed dose of meds, another by a glass of wine. This one really hurts Alan, since he really misses a nice glass of wine and the occasional beer. The third seizure was strange, as Alan had to call me when his left hand got stuck on his left leg and he couldn't move it. He forgot to take his drugs immediately so the seizure was advancing by the time I reached him. Each seizure sets him back quite a bit.

Sandy the 20-year-old cat went out in the sun during March break and never came back. Either the birds drove him insane or he drifted off under a tree somewhere. Perky now rules the house with total control having driven off the offending feline. He acts a bit like a dwarf eagle. He and Pearl, the female, appear to be setting up housekeeping in the space on top of the medicine cabinet. The two of them hide there and when you walk into the bathroom they pop up their heads and squawk. So far, it hasn't caused a seizure in any of us!

The eight fish have been interesting, too. Our fish are named after family members. There was a time when three daddy fishes died in a row, so we stopped calling anything Daddy fish (bad karma). Recently I was summoned to the basement by two frantic girls, who informed me that Andrew-goldfish was swallowing Sarah-algae-eater. I asked, "How much is still sticking out?" and was told that the tail was still showing. Using my trusty Swiss army knife and the tweezers from it, I held Andrew-goldfish in my left hand and forcibly extracted Sarah-algae-eater with the tweezers in my right. Andrew-goldfish looked quite relieved to have this thing out of its throat but, sadly, Sarah-algae-eater had suffocated in the meantime and was flushed. A short trip to the pet store and another six dollars later, we had a bigger fish to replace the flushed version.

The plan for Alan is to have an MRI in about a month. If the tumour is stable, we'll begin reducing the Tamoxifen to give Alan a better quality of life. He sleeps so much that he really isn't part of the family at all sometimes. We hope that reducing the Tamoxifen will mean he is less sleepy and a bit brighter. The anger that was so prevalent at last report seems to be easing for the moment. He is still short-tempered but not as likely to swear at any of us.

I bought him an adult tricycle and he is learning to control it. The first few times out, his weak left side caused him to crash into the snowbanks that remain at the side of the road. The last few times it has been a bit better, although last night I had to tell him to stop driving down the middle of the road when there is opposing traffic. I suppose that is the best illustration of his personality right now. He is very focused on his own desires, and if he wants to drive down the middle of the road, well then, look out, all you cars.

This also means that at all-you-can-eat meals and buffet wedding receptions he will fill his plate three or four times and then look for the next course and wonder why I keep giving him wife eyes – you know, those so-called hidden signals between a wife and a husband, that every other wife sees and the husbands don't.

The goal now for us as a family is to focus on quality of life rather than treatment. The illness is under control for now and we will try to take a breather from cancer for a month or so. Of course, it's easier said than done, because it's here and its symptoms are here.

Moyra

Every once in a while, I went off the official record and shared some of my deeper concerns with a close friend. These concerns were very personal and, in many ways, selfish, because they were about me, not about Alan and not about my children. While I was fighting for Alan, I dreaded the idea that I might have to live this way indefinitely. Rationally, I knew that I would find a way, but it was still troubling.

Tuesday, April 4, 2000 – Moyra, to a friend

I'm frazzled but hanging in. I suppose above all else I'm lonely. Most of the academic colleagues in my age group have left for greener pastures. The financial squeeze from higher up drove others from my hiring tier to other places. I also miss the man I used to have as a husband, and sometimes I'm not so sure about this one. There is a substantial change in personality that we are learning to cope with. Sometimes I see my old Alan but when he tells me to screw off, for example, it's a tricky spot to be in. For all the ups and downs in the 20 years of marriage before this, he never spoke to me the way he does now. (That isn't to say he does it daily. My mother's experience with Dad's Alzheimer's gives me a wonderful role model, but it also scares the heck out of me.)

I've spoken to some other spouses of people with brain tumours, and what he has is very normal. In some respects, I dread living with this for an indefinite period. Somehow, at some point, we will have to adjust and get past it. His therapist tells me it is not going to be an easy thing to get through if it is organic in nature. In other words, if the doctors removed the civility-grey-matter, then it's gone for good, unless other parts of the brain can be trained. I find he makes a tremendous effort when he's out in public, especially with friends and family. But when we get home, the effort is too much to maintain and he slips both physically and emotion- ally. Oddly, he is very caring and loving in the post-seizure period. It's when he is healthy that it gets tough, because he thinks it all ought to get back to normal and the rest of us are still stumbling along.

However, the anger seems to be lessening. The biking seems to be helping both emotionally and physically although it took most of my weekend to adjust the bike to his specs. Carolyn tossed out her training wheels this weekend, so the two of them can now go around the block together. It's hard on Alan to realize how much he has lost, and to see how easy many things are for me. It makes no difference to him that I have a degree in mechanical engineering. He just figures he ought to be bigger, stronger, smarter, faster, taller and higher than I am. After all, that is how he perceives it used to be, and I married him knowing that he felt that way but understanding that he did respect me for my abilities. Alan was always a bit of a dichotomy. He felt that his own work was largely inadequate, but that it was superior to everyone else's.

In any case, there you have it. Thanks for listening. I know you're out there and I am finding my way through this slowly. As I've said before, I wonder sometimes if I will come out of this with me intact, but I'm not the first, I won't be the last and it's only late at night when I've made three dozen cupcakes for Andrew and Carolyn's school that I allow myself a moment of self-pity.

Tomorrow is another day and the kiddies turn six. Wow, I made it through that didn't I? This time six years ago I was as big as a house, couldn't breathe for babies in my lungs and didn't know that three hours of sleep in a row was doing really well.

Moyra

Tuesday, May 9, 2000

Alan has been having a lot of seizures lately, including one yesterday, so we have been waiting for news on the MRI with some concern. However, the news is good. The tumour has actually become smaller for the first time, and its maximum dimension is now 2.5 cm. That is the good news! There is some concern now about the lateral ventricles, which are dilated, and something is showing in the brain stem that is probably an artifact of the MRI but will be watched just the same. It is possible that fluid is building up and causing the seizures. We now begin adjusting drug doses again to try to reduce the amount of water he is retaining.

It has been a long haul to get to this point. I feel profoundly exhausted and rather numb, but we can now look forward to a better summer than we anticipated.

For those of you who follow our continuing pet sagas, you will be sad to learn that Perky, the male bird, flew the coop the other day when the door was open for duct cleaning, leaving behind three unhappy children. We have been joined by another bird, Smokey, who was lost and needed a home. Pearl was quite upset to have lost her first mate, but seems to have adjusted to this fellow and allows him to come close. Our expected eggs-cum-science experiment will have to wait until the new fellow is fully accepted. He is doing his best to be appreciated – "see my lovely crest, see my beautiful wings."

We will try to focus now on continuing to improve Alan's quality of life. He needs to start sleeping less and he needs to have fun in some way other than sneaking calls to Lee Valley Tools and ordering up a peck of stuff. He has had enough energy to take his trike out a few times, so that is a good sign. I have this rather fantastic image of him having a seizure while on the trike, but I try to not worry too much when he goes out on big roads.

Moyra

Wednesday, May 24, 2000 – to local friends and family

I would like to ask those of you who take Alan out every so often to add salt to your list of "Alan, should you…?" topics. I was pretty sure there was a link between his leg edema and his seizures. He stopped having the seizures recently when I unmercifully cut back the salt (I am a terrible wife). He also took Furosemide, a diuretic, to reduce fluid retention. The diuretic has the fun side effect of dizziness, so it's better to avoid salt if he can.

On Monday, Alan had a great time at the family BBQ and fireworks. As some of you noticed, he ate well and kept going back for more chips and Cheezies. He also consumed about six canned drinks. Needless to say, he was puffy on Tuesday and had a Furosemide. He ate more salty stuff Wednesday when I was at work and took another diuretic, but it was too late and he had a seizure last night. It wasn't too bad, but all these things set him back. I'm trying to switch him to sugar, but he really likes salt. We are using salt substitutes, of course, but there is really nothing like a big bowl of salty-buttery popcorn.

He is rather peed-off at me right now, because salt was the last fun thing on his list.

Moyra

Wednesday, May 31, 2000

We have another MRI in a few weeks and we'll know a lot more then about the ventricles and brain stem dilation. Within the family, though, there is a sense of weariness at living this way, always waiting for the next shoe to drop, rarely sleeping the way one ought to – combined with the pleasure of having this time together.

Alan is doing quite well but gets frustrated easily with the kids, his own difficulties and me. For some reason, he and Sarah clash regularly. I guess it's a combination of pre-teen hormones and a tired-of-being-ignored dad. Carolyn told Alan the other day, "You never smile, Daddy, and you always have an angry face." Andrew is very attached to me but is willing at least to stay home with his dad rather than go shopping. Clearly, shopping is a chick thing; the guys prefer to stay home and watch television.

It takes Alan longer to do everything than he expects. Tying a tie properly takes an incredible effort. Simply getting dressed in the morning is an hour-long event. His balance is only so-so which means that a simple thing like weeding the garden is frustrating for him. He has learned to sit down while pushing the hoe around. He is enjoying the sunshine, though, and has had the bike out a few times.

His doctors are very impressed. One has said, reading between the lines, that "he doesn't understand why Alan is still with us." Another said just today in an e-mail to me, "Things are going well, surprisingly well." However, the research shows that these tumours grow resistant to Tamoxifen over time and tend to return very aggressively.

Alan's double vision has resolved itself, finally. He had some bad falls when he had dizziness and double vision. When there are two or three handles, it's hard to know which one to grab. It's amazing what adding one drug can do to the mix. The vision problems started when we added a diuretic to reduce edema at the same time as reducing the steroid. Since he bruises easily (from the steroid), he now has about six saucer-sized bruises on various parts of his anatomy in yellow, purple, red and blue. It looks a bit like I clubbed him with a baseball bat. The one on his behind is the biggest and most impressive. That's the one that happened when he fell in the closet and broke the shoe rack as he came down.

It was during this time that my own doctors put me back on anti-depressants, since I was throwing up and dropping pounds again. I knew I was in a bad place when I tried to go to a presentation in Maine. I waited all day at Dorval airport as flight after flight was cancelled due to bad thunderstorms in the States. Eventually, I gave up and went to a hotel and was in a deep, wonderful sleep within minutes. I stayed that way pretty much for sixteen hours. I truly thank the cousin who became mum for a day. I am feeling quite a bit better right now than I did a month ago. I had let myself fall back into the trap of working late into the night and on weekends on my research and writing the paper for July. Clearly, my body and mind are not willing to go to that effort yet. It worries me, because research is an essential part of being a professor. I will try to keep it going, but my production level for putting out published papers is taking a beating. These kinds of illnesses do, though, give one pause for thought about what is really important in life.

On the bird front, the new bird has mated with our female. I can tell you with considerable authority that cockatiels sing quite beautifully while mating. We are now awaiting eggs. The mating was witnessed by the children, which meant that the anatomy of mating needed to be explained to the six-year-olds. Sarah had already had the talk. At the end of a rather short but correct explanation, Andrew offered the following, "So if the birdies don't snuggle enough, the daddy stuff doesn't get to the mummy stuff and the eggs won't hatch into babies." I was at that point quite pleased with my explanation until Andrew then said, while touching a pointing finger to his arm several times, "Our teacher said all that had to happen was buzz, buzz, buzz." We assume the results of the "buzz, buzz, buzz" will appear soon because the male bird is quite serious about guarding the nest box and huffing and puffing at us when we get close. This, combined with the female bird's house-cleaning efforts of throwing pine chips out of the nest box with a disgusted look on her face, suggest things are moving along.

I have a very distinct memory of enthusiastic housecleaning on my part at the end of my own pregnancies. In those times, Alan learned to stay clear of my cleaning rag; the male bird likewise stays out of reach when the female is tossing wood chips about. He is a very attentive mate compared to Perky. It is sweet to see him groom the female, until she bites him for getting too familiar. The neighbour's cat is fascinated by the bird sounds that come from our house, and spends time at the front screen door listening and sneaking in whenever the door is open for more than a few seconds. He is a rather prodigious hunter, so we have to catch him quickly when he does get in.

Alan is planning to head off with his folks for a five-day cruise on the Rideau Canal. (The cruise boat is trapped in the Trent-Severn system and can't clear a bridge in order to get to the Rideau system, so they're waiting to see when they can leave.) After our European ODDYsee last fall, I can understand why they are avoiding airplanes. Alan is quite looking forward to the outing. I suspect he is planning to gorge on salt-laden foods. The no-buzz beer on the cruise is 0.9 percent rather than 0.5 percent, which he normally has. We tried one of those at a weekend event and it seemed to be okay. However, Alan did get ticked off when I kept dumping his wine glass, which the waitress kept refilling, into my ginger ale (ruining it!). Finally, I got up and quietly told the waitress to stay away from our end of the table. I suspect Alan is still wondering why she never came back to fill up his glass again.

July will take us to Newfoundland, where I will present a paper. We will once again build in a vacation of sorts. I will find out whether I can drive long distances with three kids and Alan in the car together. We now have Walkmans for each of the children. A recent drive to our cabin was a challenge, with Andrew singing his ABCs, Carolyn singing "C-H-I-C-K-E-N, that's the way you spell chicken," Sarah singing yet another melody and Alan listening to CBC all at the same time. I had quite a headache when we arrived at the lake.

Moyra

During the 1999–2000 academic year, I was very fortunate to be on a regularly scheduled sabbatical. I was able to continue my research program from home on a fairly active basis, making substantial changes to the software we had developed, which was now mine, and presenting my new work and our common work in thermal-mechanical analysis at several conferences. Still, I was losing contact with our overseas research collaborators and co-authors and others in the technical research community who were interested in this field. Alan would contribute from time to time in a general sense, but no longer wished to participate actively. I missed him and the partnership we had forged over the years. That part of our relationship was changing very quickly.

Once my sabbatical was over and as Alan's illness progressed, I knew I would not be able to find the consecutive hours of concentration that were required to do this research. I needed to be realistic about what I could accomplish. Once again I needed to respond to circumstances beyond my control and make a shift in my career. As the principal breadwinner and the principal caregiver of the family, I needed to be pragmatic. I struggled with my academic self, trying to determine what was meaningful, what I could contribute and how I could possibly do it. When the NSERC-Nortel Ontario Chair for Women in Science and Engineering with understanding and kindness offered me a position as her Associate Chair to help organize a number of events, such as the 2002 International Conference of Women Engineers and Scientists, I gratefully accepted. In addition to my technical research, I had maintained a small parallel research stream in this area. It was a natural fit, an opportunity to make a contribution; it gave me a reduced teaching load, which would provide some much-needed flexibility in my life, and the work itself could be done on a very flexible basis. It was the right choice and the right time, but I also knew that it could affect my long-term technical research objectives.

Tuesday, June 20, 2000

Another MRI, another three hours in waiting rooms, but Alan's tumour has not grown this cycle. You may recall it actually shrank last time, so I guess we have achieved whatever the high-dose Tamoxifen can do.

He has been having more seizures, usually one per week. They are fairly mild but involve a long recovery period in which he won't listen to me at all. You might ask what has changed, but it's critical he listen to me then because he is prone to using power tools and thinking he can fly along with other superhero antics in these periods. In any case, the doctors have added a third anti-convulsant to the mix. We used it before to control some left-side epilepsy-like behaviour, and it's unpleasant. We will try it at night so that he sleeps then, rather than adding more sleep to his already sleep-filled days. Seizures are no good at all, though, and have been hard on him since I become his mother not his wife and his nurse rather than his partner, and I'm a nag to boot.

He had a great Rideau River cruise with his folks and gained about 7 pounds in five days. His low chemo weight is gone and he is now creeping past 180 pounds (up 15 since Christmas). On the cruise, the staff cater to the elderly and those with disabilities; Alan added meeting the needs of people with terminal brain cancer to their repertoire. The staff were all over him like flies on honey. He had a great time.

This weekend a colleague visiting from Europe came to the lake and helped out. He assembled a BBQ, and then watched nervously as I tested it for leaks and turned it on. He then gleefully boiled several pots of hot water on the side burner, muttering about getting one for his summer house. On Sunday he helped me with our new easy dock. It's an aluminum dock, expensive but light enough for a wife and a kid to handle (in my dreams). The first try, in the rain with very cold lake water, was a bust. The dock is in but our friend says it looks like Belgrade after the bombing. I think it looks more like a sick creature with legs sticking out at all angles and the end under water rather than above, the latter being more traditional, I believe.

I think the problem is that the water at the end of the dock is over my head. It's tricky to carry a dock into the water, insert the legs and drop them down while simultaneously treading water or, alternatively standing on the bottom under water not breathing while holding up the dock with the left hand and then reaching up with the right hand to insert the leg through the support and then attaching the foot one-handed and lowering it to the lake bottom. Alan hates watching this kind of stuff now; it makes him feel horribly helpless. I have big plans for this weekend to get the legs upright and the planking on.

Alan had a seizure in the car on the way to the lake. He was then in recovery mode arriving at the lake insisting he could walk without my help. He fell and gashed his leg big time. He fell again later, but there was no new damage. His left leg is bruised from knee to ankle and he has a mighty gash at his shin. He was not too happy when I told him I would use rubbing alcohol to disinfect it (yow!). It needed a pressure compress for the first 24 hours and even with that it continues to bleed. The doctor added antibiotics to the mix so he doesn't get some neat germ growing in there with the trapped dirt (and, yes, his tetanus shot is up to date).

Newfoundland or BUST begins July 1.

Moyra

Friday, June 23, 2000

As you know from earlier this week, Alan is doing relatively well, although he has a dreadful cold right now. The first few cycles of chemo permanently damaged his immune system, so everything is slower to get back to normal. Several of you have asked about the gash in his leg. It is also slow to heal and is still oozing fluids and blood. This is a side effect of the Tamoxifen, which is designed to interrupt the blood supply to newly growing and dividing cells, and from the steroid, which reduces platelets for clotting. His bruises from the fall are developing beautifully. It's clear to me that he came close to breaking something, because his foot is now purple in the same way my foot was purple when I broke it years ago and the same as my ankle when I broke it last year. Over the long term, steroids weaken the bones, so he is at higher risk for fracture.

I asked the doctor about wearing compression stockings to reduce the edema in Alan's ankles and he thought it was a great idea. Alan now wears knee-high socks to improve the circulation. They seem to help and they look fine, since they are black, not the ugly flesh-coloured ones – very military, in fact.

I have purchased two new helpers for the dock installation: Jack 1 and Jack 2. We'll try them out this weekend. The forecast is for rain, of course, for Sunday. In my experience though, these guys don't mind the rain and cold.

Pearl laid an egg last evening. Both birds have retreated to the nest box and hardly stick their heads out except to attack us when we get too close. The kids are thrilled to bits and I am looking forward to being a grand-bird. I figure we've got five or so eggs to go (most cockatiels lay six in a clutch), 20 days of brooding, 21 days of screeching baby birds, and then fledging.

Tonight, ten Grade 5 girls will join us for Sarah's birthday sleepover. I will throw food down the basement stairs to the family room to feed the beasts.

Moyra

Monday, June 26, 2000

We left home Sunday morning for the lake in a downpour that flooded a good chunk of Ottawa. I had the canoe on top of the van and figured, if need be, we could paddle home. I was delighted to find out that I am now strong enough to hoist the canoe onto the van by myself. You should see my biceps. They remind me of my days in track and field, when we did weight training.

Alan was very anxious to have the canoe at the lake so he could paddle about. I'm still thinking about that one. If he can't make a rowboat work, how will he ever manage in the canoe? On the other hand, it's next to useless sitting at home. In a few years, Sarah will be sixteen and bringing dates to the lake. At that point, a canoe will be needed for long, sunburning paddles.

I was sure I would be fighting with the dock in the rain but, to my delight, the sun came out and it was hot. The kids swam around and had a gas and I brought the two new men in my life down from the car. Jack and his brother other Jack are two beautiful red guys, albeit a little short for dancing; they are only three and four feet tall. They're attractive fellows and do exactly what they're told. The rocks, mind you, were hungry and removed a few pieces of flesh here and there. I've got some bruises to prove I'm a real engineer and not just playing with neat toys.

It took a bit of work, but I jacked up the dock, left then right then left and right again, and got the shallow-water legs just about right. Then I hopped in the rowboat at Alan's suggestion and played with the deep-water legs. A couple of cycles round and round, and it looked fairly good. When I put down the plank platforms – they are about 60 pounds each and there are six of them – it shifted and heaved a bit, so I used the jacks again to move the deep-water legs. It looks pretty good although it's a bit unstable on the deep-water end. The legs go down about six feet below the water, so it's a bit like being on stilts. There is a deep-water stability kit but it has to be installed out of the water, so we'll wait until next year for that.

My next project after the Newfoundland trip is to get better steps from the car to the cabin for Alan. He is quite a bit weaker than last year and has a great deal of trouble on uneven ground. He finds also that he gets winded just going to the water and back. I find it troubling that the tumour is smaller and yet he is weaker and having more difficulty than he did last summer. Clearly, the steroids are weakening his muscles, as we were told would happen after a few years of heavy use of this drug type. (By the way, these are cortical steroids, not the anabolic steroids used by athletes cheating the system.) He really hates being weak like this and I think finds it very hard to see me able to fill in the gaps for the most part. I'm still too darn short to do some of the work, but that is why I stopped being an athlete 20-odd years ago and took up this engineering stuff.

Moyra

By now, I knew that travelling by plane under tight schedules was no longer possible for Alan. Nevertheless, I wanted us to continue to do things as a family and find the little escapes from the stress that adventure provided. The trip to Newfoundland gave us an opportunity to travel as a family and it was flexible enough that I could adapt our plans as needed. We stopped frequently at parks and picnic sites so I could rest and the kids could burn off a little energy. I bought a new camp stove that was safer for Alan to use than our older one. This meant I could snooze in the van while he made coffee for me. It felt, at times, just like other trips we had taken before. It was a good feeling.

Monday, July 17, 2000

We made it to Newfoundland and back in seventeen days! We missed several ferry rides and dealt with Alan's two seizures and some really bad edema in his leg, but we had a great time. The kids prefer expensive hotels and upscale Bed & Breakfasts to motels.

One B&B in Newfoundland took us in on the condition that we join their family party. The kids had a fantastic time singing and dancing and chasing the dog. Alan ate like a horse. By the time we left, all the guests were hugging and kissing us goodbye.

I will always hold a special spot in my heart for the school teacher who ran this Bed & Breakfast in the summer and had the kindness, even with a family party going on, to give us a big room. She was another of the earthly angels we encountered on our journey with this disease, and her hospitality was extraordinary. She showed the children games on her home computer and gave them free rein to play and explore. Her party guests and family treated us as if we were part of their family. They took over the care and feeding of Alan, just as if he were their own brother. There was Celtic music; there was laughter; there was feasting; there was good-natured teasing. It was truly a Newfoundland "time," and I will never forget it.

In Guernsey Cove, Prince Edward Island, we rented a cabin. The people there insisted we share in the steamed mussels and fresh strawberries. Andrew wanted to adopt their dog. At Encouter Creek, P.E.I., the kids played for hours in the water park and were dragged away by M.O.M., the meanest of mammals.

At Parlee Beach, New Brunswick, we saw the wedding of Michele and Ben. They were total strangers to us but the wedding looked like fun. At one point, the groom, wearing a black tux, took off his shoes. So did his bride and they walked barefoot on the beach with their attendants.

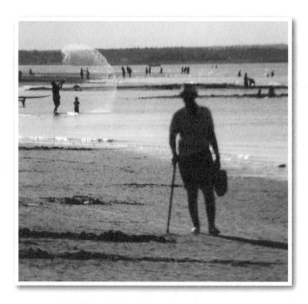

AS THE SUN BEGAN TO SET AT PARLEE BEACH,
NEW BRUNSWICK, ALAN STROLLED ALONG THE SHORE.

On the downside, Alan had back-to-back seizures in Port aux Basques, Newfoundland. They were mild but put him out for 24 hours. However, the waves were so big and the fog so bad that the fast ferry was cancelled. We took the slow boat back the next night instead, so Alan was able to sleep off the seizures without me dragging him about.

Alan has had a rough time the last few days. His ankles and feet look as if they would pop if I stuck a pin in them. Clearly, car drives are not good for his edema. He is also very stiff and has trouble getting up and about. Last year, before chemo, he played with the kids on the beach. This year he mostly slept on the beach or waited for us in the car. I think it was hard on his soul.

Alan has been struggling emotionally these last few weeks. He has shed many tears. Some of it is the drug, of course. (The Tamoxifen, in particular, is known for causing mood swings and menstrual irregularities. Alan has some of the former but none of the latter, thank heaven.) Some of it is accepting his new reality.

His anger is easing off, but his temper flares at the worst times and his choice of words can be a problem. Sarah still is the most frequent target and has the best memory for insults. Unfortunately the children have heard themselves called impediments to enjoyment and obnoxious brats. The latter came on the heels of several couples telling us that the children were marvellously behaved and so good in the bed and breakfast and at fitting in. A few days ago, Alan told us that we treated him like dog shit. When he says these things he really does feel that way. Afterward, of course, he tries to correct the hurts, but it's very hard and children are very sensitive. There is little that can be done to help him cope. His therapist gives him techniques, but he has to remember to use them.

Short-term memory is still a problem. We all went to see a movie last weekend. He decided to go alone to his choice of movie rather than see something the kids wanted to see. He was puzzled by the fact the girls wouldn't join him (Andrew had his heart set on *Pokémon*). He had completely forgotten that he had refused to sit with us at the Christmas movie and that the kids still remembered that and everything that went with it. The girls just wanted to stay with me and avoid the problems. It's very hard for him to see beyond himself – a natural consequence of his disease.

We are now looking for a pooch. Yes, a small, well-trained dog. Andrew wants a male to even things up. I have set the condition that this dog must need a home. Andrew, in particular, seems to need the companionship of a dog. He loved all the dogs we met on our trip and spent many happy moments just sitting stroking a big Newfoundland dog, a bischon friese, and a lab mix. He finds the three baby birds absolutely fascinating as they come out of the naked, ugly phase and enter the spiky new-feathers phase. However, they are not that cuddly.

Moyra

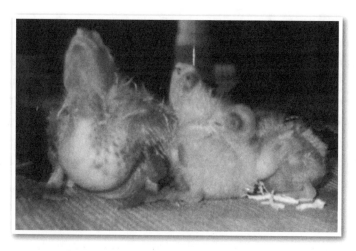

NAKED BIRDS: BIG (WITH A CROP FULL OF FOOD), MIDDLE AND LITTLE,
SITTING ON A PLACEMAT AT THE DINING ROOM TABLE.

After leaving for Newfoundland with four eggs in the nest, we returned to three newly hatched chicks and one dud. The presence of these wee creatures in our family was wonderfully soothing. They were a huge hit with the children, who named them Big, Middle and Little from a math computer game that Andrew and Carolyn enjoyed. Middle could hold his own against Big, but Little was having trouble getting enough to eat from the parents, who fed the loudest and biggest beak first. None of us was in the mood for more sadness, so the children and I agreed to help Little out. Four or five times a day, I would fill him up with a supplement using a syringe. It took some time to fill him up. Often Big and Middle would be getting cuddles at the same time and tended to scream for food as well. Big became adept at sucking back a syringe full of food in a matter of moments. In the end, all three were partly hand raised and therefore very affectionate with their human flock. Little, being the most in need, became the most attached to me and the children, and, in the end, was the most colourful of the three, with a delightful bright yellow crest.

Over the next few months, Big, renamed Jimmy, was given as a birthday present to one of Sarah's friends. Middle joined a family who had cared for Perky at one time. Their little girl referred to all cockatiels as Perkies. Little stayed with us the longest but eventually became the pet of a little boy who was a friend of a friend.

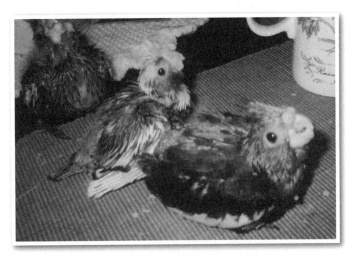

MIDDLE, WITH A DISTENDED CROP, LITTLE AND BIG,
ALL WITH FEATHERS, ON THE DINING ROOM TABLE.

August 16, 2000

Alan has had a difficult month since we returned from our trip. His problems are both emotional and physical. He has been fighting fairly significant edema (water retention), particularly in his lower legs. The diuretics he is on help but do not solve the problem. Removing salt from his diet helps the edema, but then his food, from his point of view, tastes like cardboard.

On the emotional side, he has been discouraged by his lack of ability in things such as sailing – a favourite activity – and rowing in the rowboat, a poor substitute for the canoe but at least a watercraft. On the sailing side, he discovered that he can no longer hop into his parents' sailboat and probably hasn't got the strength to control the tiller in any kind of wind. Getting into and out of the rowboat has become equally difficult. When we paddled out to the island at our lake he got into the rowboat not too badly, but generally fell, crashed or stumbled out. After a swim (life jacket mandatory), he first couldn't get out onto the rocky shore and then couldn't get back into the rowboat. It took all our combined engineering training (moments, forces, rotations) to get him onto a rock, and then all my strength to get him over the side of the rowboat without dumping the thing. Very discouraging.

When I then went off and had bags of fun sawing down trees to make a view of the lake for him, he had had enough. Today, I realized just how down he was when he declined my offer to take him into work to hear a seminar on welding. He said simply, "I'm retired." However, family members took him to lunch today and he's out for a movie this evening. Maybe that will help.

Now that Big, Middle and Little are fledging, the adult birds are at it again. This time Andrew watched the entire proceedings with interest and concluded to me, "Mummy, that looks like fun." Personally, I would find the balancing act involved in bird pairing a bit challenging. I suppose it might be okay for high-wire artists. You would think that feeding three adult-sized babies would give Smokey and Pearl pause for thought about doing it all again so soon. Certainly, twins took our minds off that sort of thing for a fairly long time. Having the birds has been a fascinating science experiment for us all, although Alan is still prone to commenting on the quantity of bird poop (he uses the other word) produced by five birds, two of which are free flyers. We are still delaying the dog arrival day by telling the kiddies that all the baby birds must have homes first.

Carolyn has become my Daddy-watcher and reports to me on all the things he shouldn't do. After a five-minute seizure earlier this month – yes, it was a long one but not too serious, as he didn't lose consciousness – she was particularly vigilant. As I did the dishes, I heard her say, "Mummy, Daddy is walking down the hall. His underwear are up but his pants are not. Is that okay?" Clearly, the short-term memory thing is still a problem. Years of training lost; the toilet seat is being left up again. (However, I'm grateful he got the underwear up.) Another time, she ratted on him when he was eating dill pickle chips. "Mummy, Daddy is eating chips. Is that okay?" "Mummy, Daddy is using the big saw. Is that okay?" It's nice having a spy in the house.

WARNING: Do not read the next paragraph if you are sensitive to "body issues."

For the pièce de résistance, Alan has a bit of a hemorrhoid problem just at the moment. I suggested that he wear feminine protection so that he wouldn't have to change his jockeys as often. After a pause for thought, some face twitching and a lot of giggles by both of us, he left the room. He returned a few minutes later and with a pained expression remarked, "It's kind of important to get that little adhesive strip on the right side, isn't it?"

Moyra

Tuesday, August 22, 2000

We are five days short of the second anniversary of our new life, and the news is good – no growth in the sucker. We will try again to reduce some side effects of the long-term use of the drugs. We now have a free-standing trapeze in the bedroom so he can pull himself up in bed at night. This will reduce the number of accidents caused by legs that can't move fast enough when required to get to the toilet because of the diuretics. It sure looks strange having this contraption in there. It was expensive, too, and is not covered by either my health plan or Home Care. More research is needed to figure out how to get around that one. In the meantime, it's ours and it's ugly but useful.

While my private insurance covered a number of things, it did not cover many very useful aids that allowed Alan to live more comfortably and with a better quality of life. I frequently reached into our savings to make it possible for him to have things like the adult tricycle, the trapeze for the bedroom and, later, an electric wheelchair lift so he could get into the house when he was unable to climb the front stairs. Each provided him with just a little more independence than he had otherwise had at the time.

I said to the oncologist, "If he is not getting worse, why is he getting worse?" The continued cognitive losses, such as having trouble recognizing his son when confronted by two small blond boys, and failing to respond to simple things, are very disturbing to us all, although Alan rarely knows he has done them. The doctor says the effects of the radiation can continue for up to two years before cognitive damage reaches the maximum, and tumours often change and grow without appearing to change, and this is very likely in his case.

In addition to the pull-up trapeze, we are now the proud owners of a handicap sticker for the car. This one really bugs Alan, but he is the one who asked for it, since his legs are so weak some days.

Moyra

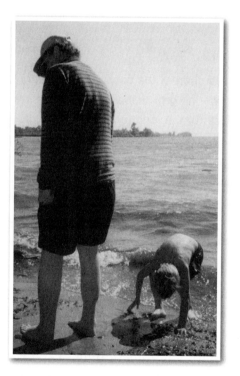

ALAN AND ANDREW AT A SMALL BEACH. THE EDEMA IN ALAN'S LEGS IS OBVIOUS. HE HAD BEEN WEARING A COMPRESSION STOCKING ON HIS RIGHT LEG. ANDREW'S PADDLING ENDED WHEN HE CUT HIS FOOT ON A SHELL.

Wednesday, August 23, 2000

A family member asked why Alan didn't design web pages or something. I thought I had better let you all know that while Alan can, on a good day, respond to e-mail, he can't, on a bad day, make things work. He just came upstairs to complain about the Mac computer again, but the problem is not with the Mac.

He forgets that he cannot trust his instincts and therefore assumes, as he always did, that he is correct. Often, he is making simple, yet fatal, errors. Tonight, for example, he reset the Mac control panels to get to the Internet. Sarah had already reset them but Alan was not able to see that. He is accustomed to changing them, and so he did.

Anyway, he cannot design web pages or anything like that. I wish he could. If it is in his long-term memory it's probably still there, but otherwise it's a struggle for him and he hates it. His oncologist still writes on the disability insurance forms every few months, "With his disease, permanent long-term disability in all areas is to be expected."

Moyra

Monday, August 28, 2000 – Alan to Janet

Moyra's last message must have been fairly grim. Everybody is replying, like you, "Not to worry about mental deficits," as if I ever did! It's very gratifying to hear I'm an inspiration to a bunch of GBM4s [glioblastoma multiforme grade 4s]. Not to brag (OK, I'll brag just a little), but I was originally diagnosed as a GBM5. I have no idea what the number signifies, except perhaps growth rate. Some people are so damn competitive they treat life as a race and try to cross the finish line first.

Alan

Wednesday, August 30, 2000 – to friends and family

Alan is quite under the weather emotionally these days. I suppose the rotten summer weather is part of it. He has discovered the limit of his technical and physical skills and it's really depressing for him.

This weekend he fell flat on his face while walking on our property at the lake and had trouble getting up. He also had another bladder accident and was wondering out loud about how long it would be before he needed diapers. Being Alan, of course, he is always trying to get a bit more out of everything than he should by carrying a bit too much, walking a bit too far, waiting a bit too long. This is an old habit genetically linked to his dad.

So, if you have a moment to send an e-mail or call, without referring to this e-mail, of course, I'd appreciate it. Please don't all call tonight. The kids go back to school next week. I'll be working pretty much full time this year, although I do have a reduced teaching load, since I taught during my sabbatical. This means I won't be here every second day to jolly him along.

We were told at the beginning that we would not likely reach the point where the long-term effects of his medications would be a problem. We are now in the stage of this being more of a serious chronic illness than an immediately life-threatening illness. Long-term use of a number of his drugs is now causing problematic side effects.

Moyra

5

September to December 2000
DECLINE

Throughout Alan's various hospital stays, two members of the clergy visited regularly. Our parish priest, Father Jim (Anglican), and members of his pastoral care team popped in about every two weeks, and Pastor Frank (Trinity Nazarene) from the church next door was also a regular visitor.

I asked for Fr. Jim's help on one of my infrequent visits to church. Since he had baptized Andrew and Carolyn, he was already aware of Alan's position on religion. Initially, we met Pastor Frank simply as a neighbour. Then, one evening, he stopped by to talk and was quickly confronted with Alan's situation. Over time, he and Alan became friends. Sarah first and then, later, Andrew and Carolyn attended Pastor's Friendship Club on Friday evenings. This extension of the pastoral care to the family gave the children a brief time away from home and gave me a much-needed break. Since that time, the beginning of Christmas has been marked by the children's pageant at Trinity.

Alan enjoyed these pastoral visits from an intellectual point of view, but stayed with his own beliefs on life and death. Still, both men continued to be available for Alan. They talked when he wanted to listen and listened when he wanted to talk. To me, each in his own way demonstrated the highest qualities of their common calling.

Years later, I found the right words to explain what their care of Alan meant to me. The words are from Isaiah, and I heard them first in Handel's *Messiah*: "He will gather his lambs in his arm, and carry them in his bosom."

Thursday, September 7, 2000 – to someone picking Alan up for an outing

Al says 11:30 a.m. is fine. He is keen to get out with someone who doesn't constantly cue him and remind him what to do, even though the occupational therapist says I must, since it's a use-it-or-lose-it thing, I gather. You also haven't heard all his jokes a zillion times.

Seriously, he's feeling pretty awful physically and emotionally. I feel for him. I sure wish he could appreciate the children more in an active way. He recently started playing checkers with Andrew and this has been helpful. He wants to love and enjoy them; it's just that they drive him nuts.

I had to laugh the other day when he said, "When I was growing up, children did what their fathers said, no questions asked." Sure, I did; my dad was in the army! The truth is Alan didn't listen any better; at least, that's what his dad says. In fact, his dad says now that he took being a father too seriously, and would do it differently if he had the chance.

Moyra

Several members of the family and even a few friends and colleagues felt comfortable taking Alan out for a coffee or lunch or even a movie. As he sometimes had seizures while he was out, it could be a bit dicey, but Alan loved these outings and always looked forward to them. The outings and the companionship made Alan feel so much better. When he felt better, the children and I felt better, too.

Thursday, September 14, 2000

Alan had some serious difficulties last Wednesday, so I took him into emergency. He was admitted on Thursday. The symptoms were a bit like those of a stroke. He is feeling much better now. It is hard to say what's going on for sure. The CT scan was inconclusive. He is having an MRI tomorrow to see whether the tumour is growing or not. The CT shows the brain midline has not shifted but there is unclear, ugly stuff there.

Early thinking is that it is mostly brain edema (water) and can be controlled. Of course there are side effects to controlling the edema. Alan is in much better spirits now that he is up and using the walker to get around. Nothing ticks him off more than being helpless and having to ask me for help. Oddly he doesn't seem to mind being helped by very attractive nurses. I guess a guy is always a guy. I suppose it also explains why Andrew thinks his Grade 1 teacher is really special – she's attractive, too.

The biggest change in all of this is that Alan has come to realize that he is seriously ill. Sounds a bit crazy, but it's true. He has always felt that he would beat this thing. Of all of us, it was best that he felt that way. A year of treatment and then back on the road again was what he expected. Coming to grips with his diagnosis has been difficult for him. He tells me he truly understood his limits the other day when he realized his underwear had been on backwards all day.

It is standard now to put living wills and power of attorney forms on file on the oncology floor when a patient like Alan comes in. We did this legal bit for Alan two years ago and it's been sitting safely away since. This morning we were asked to clarify whether or not he feels support by artificial means includes cardio-pulmonary resuscitation (CPR). Alan asked that DNR (do not resuscitate) be added to his chart. That was a hard one to get through for me. Even though I know he is terminally ill, each step towards the end is so terribly difficult.

The oncologist assures me that we have some weapons still in the war chest. Of course, it will be Alan's decision whether to continue this war. Each battle gives more information to the next patient down the road. Already his success on the trial drugs has added to the war chest for oncology, and we're told more people are now taking that drug regime and doing better than expected.

Our last baby bird has found a home. He is the most human of the three baby birds and thoroughly spoiled by his parents, who still feed him several times a day even though he is fully fledged and perfectly able to feed himself, and by my kids who carry him under their shirts. He will make a great companion. Now that the babies are fully fledged, Smokey, the male, continues to press the issue of getting another brood in the nest before the snow flies. I laughed really hard the other night when his fun was spoiled. He starts by putting one foot on Pearl's back. If she doesn't move away, he gently puts weight on that foot and lifts the other up. The next step requires co-operation, as two tails have to establish a precise mathematical relationship for balance and control. In any case, Smokey had begun to sing (as he always does, must be a guy thing) when Pearl suddenly leaned forward and tipped him right off the front of the cage over her head. Poor fellow nearly hit the floor before he re-started his flight engines and regained proper control of pitch, yaw and roll. You didn't have to be a bird to understand the words that followed. He made it very clear that he was ticked off. She just looked over the side of the cage with her head tilted to one side and then walked away. He clucked, huffed and muttered for some time and then, half an hour later, tried the foot thing again. When she dumped him the second time he was more prepared. Today she allowed him to groom her feathers so perhaps the tiff is over.

Moyra

Monday, September 18, 2000

Alan is still in hospital. Unfortunately, his balance has not improved and he is having falls and problems such as double vision. The best guess is that it is some kind of toxic effect from his drugs. His Dilantin levels are falling, so if it's the Tamoxifen-Dilantin combination it should ease soon. I am asking for him to be pulled off Tamoxifen for 48 hours. If it were Tamoxifen, we would know within that time because it always clears his system fast.

He has been moved to right beside the nurses' station yesterday after having two bad falls in the hospital. In any case, the nurses have decided to keep him under their watchful eyes. If he needs to get up, he is supposed to ring them and not use the walker without their help. If he doesn't ring and they see him up and about, they put him back to bed. He figures that at 44 he ought to be able to use the toilet whenever he wants to. However, he has become more willing to co-operate in the last 24 hours or so, since he realized he couldn't stop himself from falling. The floor becomes the ceiling in a fraction of a second, so to speak. The nurses are amazed at how much he can eat – three formal meals plus three big snacks plus whatever friends and family bring in.

The kids are okay. It is a lot better than two years ago. Sarah is old enough to watch the younger two for an hour or so (with neighbours on call) while I visit Al. They miss him, of course, but find the hospital boring. Alan can sure agree with that verdict. I am running hard on a few hours of sleep a night but so far so good with no sudden weight loss as I've had in the previous hospital cycles. I guess one becomes better at this sort of thing in time. At least I'm not the one picking him off the floor in the middle of the night and I'm not the one limiting his salt intake.

Moyra

Tuesday, September 19, 2000

The MRI appears to be negative for growth. The detailed study is to follow. According to the oncologist, with the exception of being terminally ill with brain cancer, Alan appears to be rather healthy.

The double vision is easing today with removal of Tamoxifen from his drug regime. This is the drug that controls the tumour, though; we don't really want to remove it. The doctor asked, "Which would you prefer, broken bones from falling or brain cancer progression?" I suppose the answer might be, "Which bones and how many at a time?"

Walking is better, but Alan still needs helps with everyday tasks. He showered with two young, attractive nurses today, but sadly it didn't live up to the dreams of his teenage years. He wasn't all that keen either on the swab for Vancomycin-Resistant Enterococci (VRE), bacteria that can cause infections. (VRE can be a problem on oncology wards, since patients are immuno-suppressed. VRE swabs require ye olde "bend over and cough.") He hopes to be gone for the next round of swabs in two weeks. I can see that that sort of regular testing would be a real incentive to get home.

Moyra

Sunday, September 24, 2000 – to a friend

Thanks for your visit this morning. I'm glad you got Alan when he had brains online. It was good ammunition this afternoon when I finally trapped the weekend floor doctor and asked for changes. I think I put her off last Sunday when I said Tamoxifen was the problem. She gave off very defensive body language and refused to comment. In any case, after she left the floor three or four times, the nurses summoned her back again and she finally saw me four hours after I asked for her to pop in.

When I said I wanted to talk to her about Rivotril, a drug recently added to Al's regime, she said, "I know nothing about this drug." However, I was armed and ready and had the Canadian Pharmaceutical Society (CPS) guidelines for minimum initial dose plus the list of side effects of overdose, such as really deep sleep. Then, after listening to me again and me putting circles around his side effects visible 40 minutes after taking the drug, she decided that perhaps a new dosage scheme like the one suggested by CPS would be useful.

Heaven help the little grey-haired ladies in there who only get visits by other little grey-haired ladies. I fear for my safety in the years to come. The staff is clearly overworked. So far, I have found one big error in drug doses, several small errors in timing that matter to Alan but likely to no one else, and today I found out they missed a drug test yesterday that might have determined whether it was another of his drugs causing the problem.

Alan is getting more and more bored by the minute. He and the nurses have each taken on a special calling: they try to keep him in bed, and he tries to escape. Since he is a mechanical engineer, this is not much of a problem. However, he is still recovering from those falls and he can't yet walk unaided, even with a walker, so going to the bathroom on his own is risky at best. The doctors tell me that Al's defiance of his illness is the likely reason he is alive today. Unfortunately, the defiance also makes him a bit troublesome to care for. Twice, the nurses have found him on his way down the hall to take the elevator to the cafeteria to get food. That's when they call me in to tell me he has been naughty. I feel like the principal has summoned me about a sneaky kid.

A good nurse is necessary, and the problems tend to happen with agency nurses just in here and there. Other problems occur when he has a different nurse each night, since there is a loss of continuity of care. It was today's good nurse who, after listening to me list off symptoms, kept paging the doctor back to Alan's floor to get her for me. She would pass by the room, raise her eyebrows in question, and I would answer, "Not yet." A few minutes later, she would be on the phone. Perhaps she wanted Alan to be more able to do stuff, rather than less able!

We have also been given a bit of Home Care for when he comes home. It was hard to accept for both of us, but it will give me some security when I am at work that he is being fed lunch and watched, at least for now. At the moment, we will have two hours a day, five days a week, with the possibility of weekends, if needed. I take it as a good sign that they cannot give 40 hours a week. If they do that you know you are really sick: it means the doctors think you will move to a higher plane within nine months. You may recall that we were released into palliative, with nine months to go, two years ago.

Alan is off Tamoxifen for now. I will reintroduce it once he has stopped seeing double and having other neat side effects for a few days in a row. Just recently, he asked if I could see the toads and cats that were jumping around in the corners of his vision. I replied that usually these things are not seen in a hospital. He then commented that earlier in the day the sprinkler in the ceiling had slid across the room and he was fairly sure that that wasn't quite right, either.

Moyra

Monday, October 2, 2000 – Alan's true mood!

HI EVERYBODY,

I'M HOME SO IT CAN START RAINING AGAIN.

ALAN

This was Alan's last message to our virtual support group, but he continued to write to individual friends. During October I tried to reintroduce the Tamoxifen but it was not successful. By the time Alan made it to 60 mg/day, he had red mole-size dots that apparently come from the Tamoxifen (I called them tamox-o-dots) from his belly to his biceps, and was falling again.

That was the end of Tamoxifen. His balance remained poor but for the most part he managed with a cane. Of course, after the seizures he used his walker.

Monday, October 2, 2000 – Alan to his cousin Janet, whose friend in her tumour support group also has GBM

Looks like I'm home here for good, or for a while. Tell your friend that anger and denial are very normal. I still don't believe the tumour exists and my philosophy has always been that anything that wants to take me will have to come and get me. I can provide some advice, however. If he has a wife, he should be nice to her and try to smile as much as possible, as an awful load is about to descend on her. Many marriages don't survive the strain.

Alan

Friday, November 3, 2000

During October, Alan recovered slowly from his most recent hospital stay. He has been doing well enough, I suppose, but has gone through some rough patches, caused in part by his insistence on doing things he is not ready for.

He had one wicked seizure that reminded us all how bad they can be. He has fallen a few times doing silly things, like not using his cane or reaching out to change the radio station.

He forgot how to shut off the house alarm, which added some excitement earlier this week when he set it off taking too long to leave the house. Security called the office, the neighbours showed up and the bells rang and rang.

In terms of emotions, he has rewritten his letters of farewell to the children. It had taken a remarkable amount of courage to write them in the first place. I have to give him great credit for doing that. When the time comes, they will be wonderful things for the children to have. I suppose I ought to read them some time, but I can't look at them without falling to pieces.

I know that some of you will want to know if this means the end is near. I've no idea at all what it means anymore and have given up trying to predict or guess. I suppose it means I have reached the stage where I am sort of at peace with it and plan to enjoy whatever is left to me. This does not mean that I won't get ticked off when he misbehaves, however.

Alan seems more at ease, too. The anger at being tossed this terrible disease is fading slowly and being replaced by the feeling that it's not happening fast enough for his tastes. He still feels that the likes of mass murderers ought to be the types that get this sort of thing, not the daddy of three. He is not enjoying life all that much, but I think we can get through that, too, if he can come to enjoy what he can do instead of hating what he cannot do. He has been going to the May Court Hospice once a week. There, he can chat with other people who are sick but still have something to live for. He enjoys it and has been befriended by a former professor with some connection to the United Nations. He and Alan spend time solving the problems of the free world.

Alan is getting along much better with Andrew and Carolyn. He has been able on the whole to change from being a father to being a daddy, and reading stories and just cuddling rather than trying to impart the important lessons of life like "sit up straight," "use your knife and fork," and "say 'excuse me'." Last night, Andrew climbed up into Alan's bed and went to sleep leaning against him. That's the first time in two years that has happened. Andrew stays really cool when Alan falls. He always gets his dad a pillow and blanket and covers him up. The little guys held his hands during his last big seizure and stayed there with me. When it was over, each moved one of his legs into a more comfortable position for him.

Sarah and Alan are still at odds, but I hope that will change, too. Alan can't quite give up being father to a pre-teen whose hormone valves are starting to open and who happens to like the power of being a near-adult with morning responsibilities to get the little guys and herself off to school two days a week. (I do the other three days.)

To help me de-stress I have taken up gymnastics after nearly 25 years away from it. I take it with other aging ladies. I am the oldest and we are having a gas. I have discovered that I can still do a full straddle jump on the trampoline, with pointed toes, no less. On Wednesday night I did a full front tuck off the trampoline into a foam pit. Sarah thinks it's weird that a mum would do this, but secretly I think she thinks it's kind of neat, especially since I'm still pretty good and I don't embarrass her in front of her friends. Carolyn just loves me to bits and Andrew, bless his heart, thinks I'm the coolest mummy around. He loves to watch the old girls team flying about.

I forgot to mention that Alan is now taking a controlled substance. During the Olympics, it suddenly occurred to me that Alan could take one of the anabolic steroids that certain athletes take for muscle building, since the Decadron, which controls brain swelling, also depletes muscle mass. The oncologist thought it was a great idea; it makes me wonder, though, why I was the one who thought of it. He checked some abstracts and indeed it has been used for mice with cancer taking Decadron. So, Alan got a shot in the rump yesterday. They'll try one shot a month of long-acting anabolic steroid. We hope it will help him regain some muscle mass. One of the side effects of concern is testicular atrophy but, as Alan pointed out, they're not getting much of a workout these days anyway.

Moyra

From time to time, I needed to be away from home for things such as an overnight university field trip. On these occasions, my cousin

Marguerite would slap a cheerful smile on her face and take on the challenge – and it was a challenge. The kids missed me and things were, of course, a bit different. On one such visit, Alan had a fall in the bedroom. Marguerite was trying to hoist him back into bed and called to Sarah to see if she might help. I guess it had been a difficult evening because Sarah, already in bed and probably half asleep, declined. Alan asked Marguerite why Sarah would decline and Marguerite wisely offered that Sarah was just full of sorrow. Alan remarked that he was too and they left it at that.

Sunday, November 12, 2000

I went off on a university field trip on Thursday and Friday, with Home Care, family and friends all lined up. I got home at about 9:30 Friday night. By 10:00 p.m. we were back into full crisis mode. My silly husband decided that I was taking too long to help him up, so he stood up on his own, probably had a seizure, fell down, hit his head and shoulder hard and let fly a rather colourful group of words.

On Saturday morning, his shoulder was a delightful purple-blue-red, he couldn't lift his arm and his left side was all but paralyzed. We spent from 2:00 p.m. until 10:00 p.m. getting the usual round of blood tests, CT scan and X-rays. He has a broken collarbone and has been fitted with the requisite sling.

The doctors were all set to release him back to me when I said, "Since he can't walk to the toilet and since I work and have only fifteen hours of Home Care, what do you suggest we do for the four to six hours a day he has no help, since he doesn't really think he is paralyzed?" "Umm," said the ER doctor. "I'll call oncology." "Umm," said oncology. "He may fall and break something else if you aren't there."

So, he is back in hospital with a fractured collarbone and considerable brain edema, probably from the tumour, since there is no sign of a brain bleed from the fall. His steroid level has been raised again. We're hoping that in a few days his left side will come back online.

Time to go see the silly, grumpy one that I love, still, more than you can imagine. Mind you, I'm going to give him heck again today.

Moyra

Monday, November 20, 2000

I know many of you have been worried about what Al's current situation means. I have too. Alan is still in hospital. He is very weak on the left side. His leg is moving a bit. His left arm is just hanging around. He can go from a discussion of tertiary creep in single crystal turbine blades to confusion about the time of day in a matter of minutes. Now, if he were a professor, this would be quite normal. However, as a member of the public, this is seen to be a bad sign.

The tumour has raised its ugly head again and is growing. So, the end of the stable disease stage has been reached. We are back into growth. The oncologist is leaning towards a newish oral, home-based chemo. It appears as if the $3,000/month cost will be covered by Home Care and private insurance.

We are checking to see if a new centre of activity will allow another shot of stereotactic radiation. We are looking at additional surgery, but Alan is worried about how damaged he will be if he tries this option. He also recalls how much it hurt last time and doesn't really want to try that again (for now).

Moyra

During Alan's hospital stays, he had regular visitors, particularly his family, and from time to time his friends. His parents spent time with him almost every day, and especially in the later months, his brother Doug would drop in after work for an hour or so. Alan looked forward to Doug's visits. I was often there twice each day, sometimes in the morning, when I could catch a doctor to talk to, and almost always in the evening, when Carolyn and I would pop over to kiss him good-night. We often ended up there with his parents and would all have a cup of coffee together. Carolyn loved these visits and still remembers them. They form her strongest memory of that time. Carolyn's advice to other children in her situation is "to spend as much time with your dad as you can." Her advice to parents is to make sure that the children have that special time. Sarah and Andrew were less comfortable with the hospital and so did not join us on our nightly visit. Consequently, one of Sarah's strongest memories of Alan's illness is of me being away more than she wanted.

Thursday, November 23, 2000

Alan had something called a thallium scan yesterday. It has helped clarify the situation somewhat. There has been progression of the tumour, as you know. Unfortunately the thallium scan has shown that the progression has been into the motor strip (which controls movement). This explains the paralysis on his left side, particularly his arm. You may recall that after the second craniotomy I cleared the surgeon to go as close to the motor strip as he dared, to remove as much tumour as possible. It appears to have grown in that direction again. Damn it!

Alan starts the new, expensive chemo later today. We hope it will beat the tumour into submission and give us some more time again. Home Care has agreed to cover the cost under its new rules for limited-use drugs. Alan takes one pill, five or so mornings in a row, and then has a few weeks off and does it again. At that rate, I figure each pill costs $600. I guess if you drop it on the floor you have to find it, wash it and use it.

Alan has a list of exercises to do. I have added "smile once per day" to his list. Yesterday, he actually did it. The nurses noted that I was an athletic type. They asked if he was an athletic type.

"Nope," said Alan.

"Ah," said the nurse. "You must from the intelligentsia group."

"Nope," said Al. "Actually, I'm from the enchilada group." Get it? Hot and spicy!

With respect to gymnastics, I have regained many skills I could do at sixteen years of age. My form is rather poor – I've nearly removed my chin with my knees a couple of times – but I'm getting there. Sarah delightedly pointed out that she could do one trick with an additional half-twist. This week, the "old broads and a guy" were challenged by the Show Team (kids eight to twelve) to a handstand competition. We lost. I lost to my daughter (age eleven), another mum lost to her daughter (age eight) and all of us lost to an eight-year-old boy who must be part monkey. The gymnastics is, to my surprise, a wonderful diversion. I usually arrive there in need of sleep and a bit depressed. By the time I've done a few straddle jumps on the trampoline I feel 100 percent better. If this keeps up, I'll have to try hurdles again, although I suspect that 44-year-old knees do not do as well as sixteen-year-old knees when they hit waist-high fences at full sprint speed.

Alan sends his best to you all with his usual message of "hug your kids." This journey is taking us down roads we do not like. It does put things in perspective, though. I was rear-ended in the van a few weeks ago. There was a time when that would have made me quite ticked off. But with Al's situation as baseline, what's $800 damage to a van, especially if the person who did the damage pays for it?

Smokey the bird is still trying to get another brood started. Pearl is becoming quite an expert at dumping him off at the critical moment. I feel as if I ought to have a talk with her about her choice of birth control method.

Moyra

On November 28, we celebrated my 44th birthday in the hospital cafeteria. As Alan's illness progressed, it became more challenging to create the feeling of a normal family doing normal things. My birthday gave us a chance to go out for dinner, something we had often done in the past, even if we only went as far as the cafeteria. I took a tablecloth, cake and candles and we bought the main course. Alan's parents joined us. It was a surreal situation, celebrating a birthday in a hospital cafeteria, but it worked. It felt right. You can see Alan has chubby cheeks from the steroids and, of course, his arm is in a sling to stabilize the broken collarbone. The kids were full of beans – that was absolutely normal.

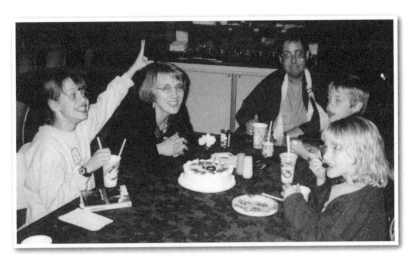

MOYRA TURNS 44!

Tuesday, November 28, 2000

Well, Alan has started the new chemo, Temodal. He actually takes 300 mg/day (three capsules, so they are only $200 each). The warnings on them are rather wild: "DO NOT CHEW, DO NOT INHALE POWDER FROM CAPSULE, IF POWDER COMES IN CONTACT WITH SKIN, WASH IMMEDIATELY."

This stuff is toxic! I'm poisoning my husband to keep him alive! Either that, or you get some wild high from it if you inhale it.

On the other hand there does seem to be continued improvement again, both cognitively and physically. Alan's left leg is much stronger and his mum and I have both noticed some returning strength in his left arm. The collarbone bruising seems to be almost gone.

This is called fourth-line chemo. In other words, this is the fourth type of chemo that has been tried. The first and best for most folks was useless for Al. His tumour grew on the first-line defence. The second and third were good for him. Now we are on to the fourth. There is not much more after this. They won't remove the tumour again, unless there is something else like radiation or chemo to follow it. I am searching for number five and may have found it, but I'm not sure it's being used in humans yet. I'm keeping the poor doctor hopping with my interminable questions.

Now for the really big news. We have a dog! Despite all my requirements, an eight-week-old puppy adopted me the other day. (I was vulnerable after long talk with Al's oncologist.) Pookie is as cute as a bug's ear, wonderful with the children and very smart.

We took him in to meet Alan yesterday. It's okay to have animals on the oncology ward; they are happy to have pets visit. The little fellow immediately crawled onto Alan's tummy, climbed to his chin, licked him thoroughly, wrestled with the sheets for a bit, chewed on this and that, and then curled up and went to sleep. Later, Alan and I went for a walk, with Alan in the wheelchair, and the dog slept in the crook of Al's arm. Alan was very pleased, although, like me, he never intended that we have a dog this small. It weighs less than 2 pounds at the moment and is a Yorkie-Terrier-Pomeranian-Poodle mix. Somebody pointed out that his rear end looks a bit like a German Shepherd's (hmmmm).

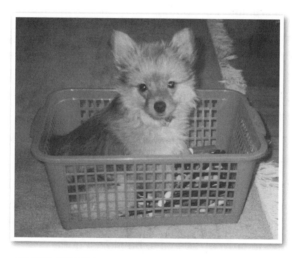

POOKIE, SITTING IN A BASKET OF MARKERS AND CRAYONS.

This dog impressed me immediately. He slept through the night on the second night home; it took my human children years to figure that out! The birds are a bit perplexed by this addition to the zoo. Pearl struts around with her wings up trying to look big. Smokey has made beak-nose contact, at which point both creatures freaked out. Pookie is very good and doesn't bark at or chase the birds yet, although he is trying hard to find the dog that lives behind the mirror. I think the best of all of this was seeing the reaction of the children, who adore Pookie as much as he adores them.

Alan has been tolerating the chemo well. We don't know when or if he can return home, but hope he will get well enough to join us for some more time at home. At the moment he can't walk or even transfer independently from bed to wheelchair, but it is coming along. He is well enough now to watch movies and has been catching up on things.

Moyra

Once again, a new life in the family immediately gave us a focus other than Alan's illness. Pookie became the recipient of the love of three children and this very tired mummy. I had seen the little creature in the pet store window shortly after speaking to Alan's oncologist, who told me that Alan had only about three months left to him. I walked by the window on the way to the bank and noticed this little dog watching me. When I passed by again he was still looking out. Later, I passed by the window a third time and he was still there and still looking out. We made eye contact. It was enough. Reacting on pure instinct, I took him home. When I arrived home and lifted him out of my coat, you could feel the family mood lighten. My instinct had been right, as Pookie instantly began to help us deal with our grief.

Even with the news about Alan becoming worse, I continued to read medical journals looking for something that might offer some sort of relief from the continued progression of the disease. I wanted to hold the door open just a little longer.

Alan was now on Temodal, and was tolerating it well, but I was still looking for medications that might help him. In my reading, I stumbled across a paper by some California researchers (in *Neurosurgery*, 28, no. 1, March 1996) indicating that people who have resistance to Tamoxifen might not have a resistance to a drug called Hypericin. I stored this piece of intelligence so I could propose it to the doctors in case the Temodal stopped being effective. As it turned out, we would use it.

As Alan's illness progressed, I realized that I should find ways to make my life easier but I didn't always know how to make that happen. The day-to-day activities were familiar and helped me to feel normal. Still, they took time away from things that needed attention. A group of friends again picked up on my inability to separate the complexities of life and illness from the very normal but time-consuming activities needed to maintain a household. They again presented me with a Christmas gift of winter snow blowing and added summer hedge trimming. I should have figured that one out on my own.

Monday, December 11, 2000 – to the friends who gave me the gift of snow-blowing service

I was absolutely stunned to find a pretty gift bag and card waiting for me today. Your gift of snow blowing and hedge trimming is so very kind. It means a great deal to me to know that so many others are out there cheering for us. Tomorrow morning, I will sip my hot coffee while the fellow outside freezes his anatomy taking snow off my driveway. Nice timing!

Alan is learning to walk again. I guess that makes it the fourth time. Each is more difficult than the last. He is in reasonable spirits and hoping to return home later this week. He will be largely wheelchair bound this time. Each step down the path becomes more limiting than the ones before. There is simply no cure for this thing. We can, at best, hope for some good time still.

I will try to take more time off over Christmas than I usually do. The social workers keep telling me to make it a good Christmas for the kids. I'm getting better at reading between the lines than I used to be, bearing in mind that two years ago they told me that Christmas 1998 would be our last together. What they don't tell me is how to make Christmas good except to build memories.

Once again, thanks so much for everything.

Moyra

Wednesday, December 13, 2000

Alan managed about 30 steps yesterday, with assistance. He is not yet able to transfer himself on his own from a bed to wheelchair, so I have asked that he stay in hospital a few more days to get that down pat.

The latest chemo seems to be working, since function is slowly returning to his left side. His leg is able to take weight and he can almost make a fist. He still can't lift his left arm. He has a senior physiotherapy student working with him every day. He is the subject of her senior thesis. She is clearly gunning for an A.

Alan was put on Hypericin (St. John's wort), which has been shown to possibly be effective in preventing growth of new blood vessels to the tumour. Unfortunately, this means he has to come off his anti-depressant, Zoloft, as one counter-indicates the other. It hasn't been fun. Yesterday, a psych-type came down and recommended that we risk the high-blood pressure and give Alan some Zoloft to control the depression. We hope this will stabilize his mood swings and anger and sadness, while possibly allowing the Hypericin to do its job.

We are busy rearranging the house for his return home in a wheelchair. We have a nifty electric lift at the front door and more space around the bed. The children have announced that the lift is too slow (i.e. no fun). I think they expected something a bit more exotic.

I did a trip to Las Vegas last week to present a paper. It went fine but my heart wasn't in it. Nevertheless, this kind of thing has to be done, I suppose. At least I got a bit of sleep, despite taking the red-eye flight both ways. There was a ticket mix-up on the way there, and to make up for it I was flown first class to Vegas, with a nice big blue leather seat, lots of leg room and pretty china. I came back with the cattle.

I found myself going through the motions of presenting the paper, knowing that it was likely to be the last time Alan's name would appear with mine. I did not enjoy that part of it at all. It forced me to recognize that there had been another fundamental and irrevocable change in our partnership.

The kids and pup stayed with friends in Windsor while I was away, so they (the kids, that is) had a break. The friends didn't have a break! Pookie the pup has been one of the smartest purchases I've ever made. He has been to the hospital (with permission), visited all kinds of cancer patients, been to the kids' school and been on the airplane, where the flight attendants went all gooey over him. The kids love him to bits, carry him around like a baby, fight over who can hold him next. All for a ball of fluff that still weighs less than 2 pounds!

I arrived home from Vegas to find that Pearl had moved on to a higher plane, and we had a moonlight graveside service that very night. What a lot of tears were shed – her death was just a bit too close to home. Smokey stood guard over her body until the burial and then called for her for several days. Now he keeps company with the pup. I wondered if this bird would learn to speak. He can. He now barks and whines like a dog! Pookie figures the bird is for chasing. The bird thinks the dog is a potential mate. Right now, one (the bird) is on my shoulder; the other is on my lap. This place is crazy!

We're hoping Alan will return home next week. I can do my exam marking at home and keep an eye on him, along with Home Care, which is still only fifteen hours a week. Alan may be able to go to the rehabilitation centre after that to improve some of his function, but with such a short life expectancy they may not accept him.

Back to one day at a time...

Moyra

Years before, when Alan and I finished our doctorates, my mother had given us the large two-volume Oxford dictionary, complete with a magnifying glass, and she had given me a brand new copy of the story *The Little Engine that Could*. When I asked why, she informed me that as a little girl I had loved that story. No doubt I had, like most children, demanded that she read my favourite too many times. Yet, the analogy to my life and how I continued to approach it was significant. I think I can, I think I can; one step at a time, one day at a time.

Tuesday, December 19, 2000

I plan to have Alan home on Thursday. He can have the pleasure of watching me mark exams for a few days. I figure after three or four days of me marking, he'll be begging to go back to the hospital. Both the quality of the meals and the personality of the cook are somewhat challenged during marking time.

The kids are looking forward to having Daddy home. I don't think they truly understand how physically disabled he is this time around. However, he is improving and once he is home without his hospital staff doing things for him, he should improve even more. I will have to see how well I respond to him ringing a small bell to get my attention.

Sarah has expressed some concern about how the two of them will get along. It is a question I ask, too. For five weeks now, she has been enjoying the rank of second-in-command. In fact, all of the kiddies have done really well. Andrew and Carolyn made me breakfast last weekend – scrambled eggs (microwaved version). They also get a real kick out of being able to do for themselves. Andrew has learned to make single-serving Kraft Dinner. I figure he is ready for university now – milk, eggs and Kraft Dinner, with an apple tossed in now and again.

Here we go again for our third "last Christmas" together.

Moyra

When I took Alan home, we received a note of instructions from the doctor on the oncology floor who was taking care of Alan's medical and emotional needs on a day-to-day basis. She knew it was going to be a rough ride because her note ended like this:

> "I hope it goes well at home, but you have the option to come directly back here until Sat. a.m.
>
> It has been a pleasure working with you … You are both an inspiration. I wish you happiness and peace."

It was a very difficult Christmas. Alan and I tried to make it special for the children, but the effort was almost too much for both of us.

I remember praying simply for the physical and emotional strength to get through it. I didn't see how the tumour could be beaten into submission yet again. After my talk with Alan's oncologist about how few months likely remained to us, I felt very much like I had now only a toe in the door that was closing.

Friday, December 29, 2000

After much soul searching and talking to Al's parents and a few medical types, I took him back to the hospital on Wednesday afternoon. It was becoming difficult to manage, especially since it was just me and his folks doing the work. It's very tricky to find even paid-for agency care over Christmas, and not one person would even consider marking my exams as well. I think we were managing about 4/10, and I see that as a failing grade. (A number of my students might beg to disagree, however.)

A few transfers from bed to chair had become lifts (and controlled crashes), and my back was suggesting that heaving a large man about was perhaps not in my best interests. The funniest ones occurred when Alan's good hand and arm would remain attached to a support rail in one room while I had his legs and tummy in another room or when the commode brakes failed and the commode shot out backwards and there were the two of us in various stages of undress, "Tower this is Air Oddy 747 heavy. Advise we will not make runway 5 east. Unable to go around. We're going down!"

This is the first time I have not just kept going forward with something and instead taken a step back. It came down to the question "Should I?" rather than "Could I?" I could have gone on, but I think it was better that I let it go this time. Carolyn tells me that Daddy is nicer in the hospital. Perhaps that is because he makes the effort for the short visits but can't pull it off when he is home all day with three kiddies who are just a wee bit excited.

Alan seems to listen better to the nurses in uniforms than he does to me. I suppose, with me, there is no more fear factor. He knows I'm a wuss when it comes to this nurturing stuff. Sure, I might grump a bit, but he just uses puppy eyes on me and I cave right in. Pookie quickly learned this cute behaviour as well; hence, middle-of-the-night visits to the toilet (Alan) and the litter box (pup) were commonplace.

Moyra

Sunday, December 31, 2000

Here are my best guesses to some of the questions that many of you are trying to ask but are dancing around.

No, surgery is not an option unless there is something to chase it with. As you know, after both resections the tumour grew from zip to 2 cm in a few weeks. With the tumour in his motor strip they won't be able to remove nearly as much. There is no new chemo at this time. Other options are pretty way out, but I am looking at them. His Karnofsky score (brain tumour IQ) has dropped a great deal and he is not eligible for a number of things since he can no longer walk. The basic requirement for many trials is that he can take care of his own needs with minimal help. There are some things that could be tried but they have to be balanced against quality of life and pain.

Yes, I have told the kids. I have said that their daddy has only a few months to live, unless the Temodal works. They were not surprised by this, and after a few tears and a long cuddle, they returned to playing. They seemed to be comforted by the idea of a heaven where the happy part of the person goes: the daddy who sailed and made sandcastles and wrestled with them, the daddy who hugged them and read them stories and walked them to school.

Yes, a new MRI/CT scan will be done. There are two reasons for the delay: 1) in the hope that the Temodal will do something, they want to wait for the effects of cycle two to show up; and 2) if the progression is there and getting worse, it will not help Alan's emotional well-being. The tumour is as big as it has ever been, but Alan has been doing better than he ought to under the circumstances.

I had to pry the numbers out of the doctors for me to know. When Alan seems impatient for the test, I usually explain that the doctors are waiting for the effect of the Temodal to show up (two cycles). If there is a positive effect, we go to three cycles.

Yes, his sense of time and reality is impaired right now. He gets names and faces confused at times, but no more than he has in the last few months. It may be the first time you have seen it in all its glory. He has symptoms of obsessive-compulsive behaviour that have been with us since the first surgery. Do not be alarmed if you find him counting things or wanting something done now. It is part of the illness.

Yes, he seems angry again. I suppose the tumour is pushing on that bit again. He also forgets his manners, and you may find him pulling down his drawers to have a poop while you are there. It's your call. Leave for a few minutes or suggest he wait until you have gone. He needs to be cued to focus. You might find he watches television while you are with him and ignores you. You might find he doesn't smile when you arrive. You might find that, after sitting with no conversation for an hour, you make it out of his room, only to have him call you back to chat.

Yes, I have his power of attorney for all things. I have not yet activated it legally, but it is getting close to the point where I may have to do that. He still has a bank card and a credit card. He is buying things from the Shopping Channel and thinking of making charitable contributions to groups that he never cared about before.

Yes, the May Court Hospice is about care at the end of life. Their goal is to make it as good as it can be with whirlpools, massage, good food and the companionship of others in a family setting.

Yes, when he makes a joke he still forgets to smile.

Moyra

6

January to March 2001
FINAL STRUGGLES

When he was home at Christmas, Alan went to the drawer in which I kept all the prayer books and bibles that had come our way through our families. He took his great-grandmother's *Book of Common Prayer*, given to her in 1933 on her 81st birthday, back to the hospital with him. Although he did not advertise the fact, he started reading the prayers in the book. Alan enjoyed reading history books: there was a historical context in this book that likely appealed to him, since the Evening Prayer section refers to King George, Queen Mary and Edward, Prince of Wales. It goes on to say, "Endue with wisdom the Governor-General of this Dominion."

I was surprised to learn that my shit-happens, there-is-no-God husband had considered prayer. We never discussed it, as I sensed he wanted to keep it private, but I hope it brought him, in those long hours when he was alone with his thoughts, some of the comfort prayer had given me, especially in the last few years. Alan marked the Prayer for All Conditions of Men using a family Christmas bookmark dated 1929. The prayer ends in this way:

Finally, we commend to thy fatherly goodness all those, who are any ways afflicted or distressed in mind, body or estate: that it may please thee to comfort and relieve them, according to their several necessities, giving them patience under their sufferings, and a happy issue out of all their afflictions.

Being ever practical and thorough in his research, Alan also marked one other section. The worn purple ribbon of his great-grandmother's prayer book still marks The Order for the Burial of the Dead.

During the late fall and after he returned to hospital, Alan had access to an occupational therapy workshop. With the help of a volunteer, he made a box that he later gave to Carolyn. He enjoyed these sessions immensely and I was very thankful for them. There was so little left in his life that he could call fun.

Monday, January 8, 2001

To the amazement of all, Alan's tumour has stopped growing again. It was about 2.5 cm to 3 cm in September with some questions about growth. Although the doctors had a general feeling that something was going on, they could find no evidence of this. He had an ugly CT scan when I took him for the fractured collarbone on November 11; they did an MRI about ten days later. As you know, the tumour was into his motor strip, but you may not have known that it was an irregular 6 cm. You did know that his oncologist told me then that Alan had maybe three months left to live.

Well, he had an MRI Thursday and it is still 6 cm. Wow. We don't know if it's the Temodal, the Hypericin (St John's wort) or both, or just blind luck. In any case, it's surprising and good news.

I have told Alan the size so he knows all the data. I had held that back before, because he hadn't asked and because the doctors were concerned about his emotional health. He spent about ten minutes holding a ruler to his head and checking it out. He was not impressed. However, he is talking about learning a new programming language.

The doctors still feel we have only a few months at best. That is not good news.

Moyra

Sunday, February 4, 2001 – to a friend with headaches

When it comes to headaches, most of them are just headaches. That's why we didn't get alarmed when the doctors said that Alan's were a normal side effect of general anesthetic or a secondary infection. When this sort of thing happens, everything makes one paranoid. Andrew gets a headache and I wonder. Of course, the last time he had a bad headache he ended up with ocular cellulitis, so I'm even more paranoid than ever.

Alan probably had more headaches the year before diagnosis than in previous years. Because he was working two contracts, we figured this was to be expected. Would it have made a difference if he had had a scan earlier? Maybe, but we'll never know. The doctor said it would have taken about six months for the tumour to grow to the original size.

Certainly, I felt something was wrong almost a year before, and even at the Christmas before, when he was dog-tired and had no energy at all.

Moyra

Thursday, February 8, 2001

There is no good news about Alan, but on the other hand there is no bad news either.

He has completed the third cycle of the latest chemo drug and is approaching the fourth. His morning headaches have returned in the last few days and that is not good, but they could be just regular headaches. It will take a CT scan to know, but there are none scheduled at the moment.

We are waiting to find a placement for him, perhaps in a hospice. Home is out of the question now, due largely to his paralysis and his temper. All of the medical-social work team now agree that the children need to have good memories of their daddy, not the memories that come with living with this disease on a daily basis. He can control things for our short visits, and that works well for the children.

He came home on Sunday for roast-beef dinner, a favourite, and it was a comedy-tragedy. It started out pretty well with the pickup, although getting into the van was a challenge. (Getting out is easier, since gravity is your friend.) At home, things went sour very fast. The winterized lift (winterized for California?) was too slippery to pull the wheelchair into it, so I pushed the chair into it.

Just as Carolyn was warning me that I was going to hit the wall at a funny angle, I did. Alan has no sense of balance, so he was unable to lean his weight the right way. Over we went from the ramp of the lift – him, me and the wheelchair but not, fortunately, Carolyn. Alan still doesn't really know that he landed partially on top of me, because he was too busy trying not to call me all the names he has learned since childhood.

Once I extracted myself, I started trying to get Alan back in the chair. Note to self: tie husband in chair next time. It was not a good day for Al's legs. With the bulk of his coat and boots, I couldn't lift him. I had to ask Sarah to get a neighbour. He came over in a big rush but he had recently had surgery on his arm and so could use only one side of his body to help me. He was wearing indoor clothes, since he had been watching football. I was now without a coat or mittens so I could get a grip on Alan. Alan was in various stages of undress, since his pants kept getting used as a point for pushing and pulling. He was wearing a gait belt which helped us lift him from the waist, but that helps only with the top half! With all of us huffing and puffing, we restored Al to the chair, got him in the lift and safely into the house. My little plywood ramps right at the door work just a treat for that and have a nice rough surface for traction.

By this time, the roast was headed for overdone, the potatoes were still in the bag, the steamed veggies were going to have to cook some other way, and my plans for homemade pie had been replaced with "What's in the freezer?"

Alan, exhausted by this simple trip home, had a rest. His folks arrived soon after we did and took over Alan duty while I attempted to salvage by divine providence a Sunday dinner.

The next major hurdle was the bathroom. Alan and I had a routine for that but his parents didn't know it and of course Alan had forgotten it.

We had another of those "you have to trust me" sessions in which Alan had to trust me not to drop him headfirst into the toilet or shower or sink. Of course, after I crashed his chair, I could understand his reluctance to let me hold him up while pulling down his pants. (As if the loss of dignity was not bad enough.)

In the end, we did have a nice visit and dinner, but by 8:00 p.m., Alan was ready to go back to hospital to get some rest and escape from busy family life. So back we went. By the time I tucked him into his bed he was exhausted. It was disappointing to him to find out that he preferred the calm, quiet care of his nurses to the hurly-burly life of clattering dishes, bath times, homework and chaos.

So we wait now for a bed at the Élisabeth Bruyère chronic palliative unit. His move there requires a change in policy, which yours truly, armed with literature on the use of Temodal as a palliative treatment versus an active chemo treatment, has initiated. We will have an interview at the unit next week, where they will explain to us what they cannot or will not do, and I explain to them that we hope Alan will have a fighting chance with this new drug, but that they are to do nothing heroic if he has a cardiac arrest or some such thing. Since Al's blood pressure and general health are excellent, major organ failure seems unlikely. In thirteen days he will pass another milestone – the three months he was given before Christmas. Of course, the Temodal was not expected to halt the tumour so effectively at 6 cm. That's my boy – one of 27 percent who shows a statistical response as opposed to the 63 percent for whom it is not useful. He now has to beat the next statistic for those for whom there is a response; the response tends to last, statistically, for only a few months.

On the home front, Pookie the dog has been a real blessing. Pookie and Smokey the bird have become friends. In the morning, Smokey swoops into my bedroom or down from his perch in my room, although he sometimes spends the night sleeping on Carolyn's shoulder (Carolyn is sleeping in Alan's bed at the moment because it makes her feel closer to him). Then, once on the bed, he and the dog wrestle! (Yes, Pookie now sleeps on the bed with me, but he is not allowed between the sheets!) Smokey spreads his wings and stomps around the bed and tries to bite Pookie's nose and ears. Pookie puts a front paw on Smokey and then attempts to put Smokey's head in his open mouth. Pookie wiggles his open mouth back and forth over the bird's head. It's clear that they love it and are playing. Sometimes Pookie's nose gets too hard a bite and he yelps, and sometimes Pookie gets too big a mouthful of bird and Smokey squawks. I wait for the day when the ratting instinct in the dog takes over and we are greeted one evening with a tricky situation.

Gymnastics is still a real hit. I can now do a front tuck in the air over the trampoline and a pike forward tuck in the air off the tramp into the pit. I am working on an L-sit on the rings, but the old abs need a bit of strength yet. We keep attracting parents who were once high school athletes, and our group is now up to eight. The day after a session, I always find muscles I didn't know I had, but it's a good workout and we laugh so hard at the antics of the others. I won the push-up contest last week at close to 20 although the last five were not military style, which is why we don't know how many I really did.

Within a few weeks, Alan will likely move to the chronic palliative care unit and we will start down another road.

Moyra

As we prepared to move Alan to the Élisabeth Bruyère chronic palliative unit, I had to acknowledge that there would be no more active treatment, although the Temodal would continue as a palliative treatment. Alan had the "do not resuscitate" notation on his file; still, we needed to establish treatment protocols for other things that might happen. Alan had made it clear to me that he didn't want to descend into some sort of earth-based hell and to please let him go if the chance came. In discussions with his palliative doctors and his parents, we agreed that any further treatment would be handled at Bruyère. Alan would not be sent back to a critical care hospital for any reason. It was a difficult decision, especially for his mother. I was grateful that his parents were willing to be part of the decision; I can't imagine how it must be to make that kind of choice for your own child. It was awful enough to do it as a wife respecting her husband's wishes. For me it was, ultimately, a matter of acknowledging to myself that I had finally reached the point at which I could stop fighting the battle. There would be no more research on glioblastoma multiforme. With profound regret, I surrendered to this disease. Once the children were in bed and asleep, I cried until I could cry no longer.

Monday, February 26, 2001

Alan will be moving to the chronic palliative unit on Wednesday of this week. As he says, it must be a pretty exclusive club, because they interviewed not only his wife but also his parents a few weeks ago. I gather we passed the exam.

It is difficult to make this move to palliative, because it is an acceptance on all our parts that a cure is no longer viewed as even a remote possibility but now is in the realm of miracle. Alan will be able to keep taking the Temodal, which seems to be controlling the tumour at the moment. I successfully weaseled them into changing the precedent for admission on active treatment. This has changed my status among the medical types at the hospital considerably. They have never met a wife-of who could pull off that sort of thing.

Alan always stood in the top few percent of our engineering class. He clearly is doing the same now. Not only is the tumour being held in check for now at 6 cm, he can stand unaided for 20 seconds or so, and he can walk about 150 steps, with only a little assistance, twice a day.

Moyra

Wednesday, February 28, 2001

Alan has been transferred to the Élisabeth Bruyère chronic palliative unit, room 509. It went fairly well, although Alan is not happy to be crossing this bridge.

Moyra

When Alan moved to Élisabeth Bruyère, the hospital first suggested that an ambulance could take him there. I declined this offer and said I would drive him myself. I knew it was the last bridge he would cross and I wanted to cross it with him. I don't recall that we talked much about anything in particular. What I remember feeling is a strong emotional connection – we both knew what this meant.

The chronic palliative unit was very quiet, and Alan and all of us missed the hubbub of the hospital, particularly in the evening. At the hospital, we usually rolled Alan downstairs to the coffee shop. He enjoyed watching the hustle and bustle, which was not unlike that of a family at the end of a day of school and work, preparing for dinner and the activities of the evening. There were people all around, at the coffee shop, gift shop and a convenience store. Just being in the centre of it made him feel that he was still part of the busy community. In the palliative unit, things were much quieter, which concerned him. The family joked that the streets rolled up much earlier there. He felt more hospitalized in palliative care than he did in hospital. However, the palliative unit did offer outings. He was looking forward to visiting the nearby Canadian War Museum and the National Gallery when the weather improved.

On Friday evening, the kids and I showed up to take Alan to the cafeteria for dinner. His brother Doug joined us. It was a good meal. The kids were happy and Alan was in good spirits. It was to be our last meal together as a family, and the last memory the children would have of their dad up and about and busy with life. The next morning he had a sore back, which he blamed on his bed. It would turn out to have a much more serious cause: a blood clot.

The palliative care team was wonderful. I was impressed, yet again, by the level of compassion in his care. As Saturday progressed, I learned more about what faced us. By coincidence, Dr. L., his therapist, dropped in. Alan and Dr. L. talked, and I know it was great comfort to Alan. As she left, I promised Alan that I would make sure there was no pain. I went home in the evening thinking that things would be okay, but late in the night I got a phone call asking me to return. I spent the early morning hours with Alan, who mostly drifted into and out of sleep but occasionally communicated by squeezing my hand. His parents joined me later.

At one point Alan was trying to tell me something, but his speech was hard to understand because he was medicated. As I kept trying to understand, he suddenly threw his good arm around me and gave me such a big hug it nearly broke my heart. He was saying "I love you" in the only way he could.

In the morning, I went home to the children. Calls were made to Alan's siblings. We had started the last day.

Sunday, March 4, 2001 (morning)

Alan has developed a major blood clot in his right lung. He came very close to death last night, but once again beat the odds. However, it looks serious. Some of you were planning to visit Alan. I think we will say it's family and doctors only until further notice.

If you pray, now is a good time to do it.

Moyra

Later that Sunday morning, I found myself in a United church listening to Sarah's choir sing in its annual guest appearance. Their young voices were beautiful and I cried again as I realized that this little girl, and her brother and sister who sat beside me, would soon be fatherless. This door was closing and I would soon be alone with my little family.

Psalm 91 was written in the Order of Service that day. I had never seen this interpretation of Psalm 91 before, but I allowed myself to be comforted by the reference to eagles. Alan loved eagles and other birds of prey, but would have insisted that it was a mere coincidence that they were mentioned on that particular day.

After choir, Andrew and Carolyn chose to go and kiss their dad goodbye. Sarah opted to go to a friend's house. She regretted her decision later, but did not understand at the time the significance of the situation.

The family stayed with Alan throughout the afternoon and evening. It was a bit of a party, in fact, with sadness and silly jokes intermingled. Al would have liked that. About 9:00 p.m., his siblings and their spouses left the room to give Alan's parents and me some time with him. His death was very simple: he stopped breathing as the load on his heart and lungs from the blood clot that had moved from his leg to his lung became too much. (I've spoken to several doctors about how a small clot becomes an embolism. It's fairly common in those who don't move around very much, especially as cancer, in general, makes the blood sticky. Since there is very little that can be done to treat it – clot blasters cannot be used due to the risk of bleeding, in Al's case in the brain – it is a matter of time and luck.)

After Alan's death, I went home to tell the children. My cousin Marguerite had been, once again, caring for them. They looked at me hopefully when I came through the door, but this time there was no good news. We sat together on the couch and I told them that their daddy's long fight was over. There were lots of tears. Later, when they were asleep, I sent this e-mail using Psalm 91, from the service that morning.

Sunday, March 4, 2001 (evening)

Alan's fight with brain cancer ended tonight. I will try to send out an e-mail about services and donations tomorrow. Alan has donated his corneas and long bones to those who might need them.

And he will raise you up on eagles' wings,
bear you on the breath of dawn,
make you to shine like the sun, and
hold you in the palm of his hand
Psalm 91

Moyra

Despite the lateness of the hour, e-mails from our friends began to pour in. Just as they had been at the beginning, they were a comfort at the end. Over the upcoming week I felt so very blessed to have such support. The children received cards and notes from their classmates. Their messages were equally sweet. I saved them all so that when the children have grown up, they will have that record for themselves.

On Monday, I made the arrangements for his service, and it was at the funeral home that I finished writing his obituary. I had not been able to face it before his death. The words "blessed by your tender and gentle care" came easily to my pen. The simple realization that we had been blessed in this way was comforting. Faces, many without names, came to mind as I wrote those words: the cheerful man who washed Alan's hospital room floor, the ladies in the cafeteria who always had a smile for the children, the volunteers in occupational therapy, coffee shops and clinics, the pastoral care teams, and the broad medical community who fought the disease with us.

ODDY, Alan Sinclair
B.Eng., M.Eng., Ph.D., P.Eng.
At age 44, after a valiant fight with cancer. A graduate of Canterbury High School and Carleton University Alan began his career at the Dockyard Research Establishment Atlantic in Halifax. He also worked at Acres Consulting Services Ltd. in Niagara Falls and was a post-doctoral fellow and employee of the Materials Technology Laboratory of Natural Resources Canada. After completing a research associateship at Carleton University he started his own company, OMNIS in 1993. Much loved husband and research partner of Moyra (McDill). Very, very proud father of Sarah, Andrew and Carolyn. Dear son of Lorna and Leonard Oddy. Cherished grandson of Lillian (the late Stanley) of Winnipeg and the late Janet and Angus Cameron. Brother of Patricia (Bruce Boyd), Douglas (Yolond), Susan (Randy Scott) and Catherine (Brian Kelly). Uncle and sandcastle builder for Brian, Alan, Steven, Tina, Cameron, Lee, Chris, Kenneth, Jeffrey, Nicholas, Scott, Samantha, Christine and Elizabeth. Friends may attend a Memorial Service at St. Thomas the Apostle Anglican Church, 2345 Alta Vista Drive on Saturday, March 10, 2001 at 2 p.m. Fellowship in the Parish Hall afterward. In lieu of flowers, for those who wish, donations may be made to Alan's special causes: The Owl Foundation, The Nature Conservancy of Canada, The Brain Tumor Association, The Hospice At May Court or the Elisabeth Bruyère Health Centre. The family wishes to thank the staff of the Ottawa Regional Cancer Clinic, The Ottawa General Campus, The May Court and Elisabeth Bruyère. Our journey was blessed by your tender, gentle care.

Hulse, Playfair
🍁*McGarry 233-1143*

———————————105551

TUESDAY, MARCH 6, 2001

ALAN'S OBITUARY FROM THE OTTAWA *CITIZEN*

Here is a very small sample of the messages I received.

I admire all that you managed to do for both Alan and the children during these last few years. Your dedication, energy and remarkable determination are truly an inspiration. Please know that you are in our thoughts and prayers (yes, we pray at night and have said special prayers for Alan this week).

*

I shall remember Alan as a charming person, a patient teacher, committed to a thorough understanding of his science (not a man to cut corners!), an effective champion, forthright with his opinions but open to discussion, creative, energetic and the keeper of an incisive wit.

*

Alan was more than a colleague to me. I appreciated Alan very much – his humour but most of all his ability to play with kids and being one with them in a natural way (some people just sound silly when pretending). A man that has contact with the child in himself is also near the kingdom of heaven (Mark 10:14).

*

We'll never get used to addressing you without Alan.
You were a brilliant couple.
We'll never get used to thinking about Alan in the past.
He was a tender husband, loving dad and a superb friend.
We will always miss him – his courage, intellect, honesty, tact and wonderful sense of humour.
He was the best member of the elite club of intelligentsia.

*

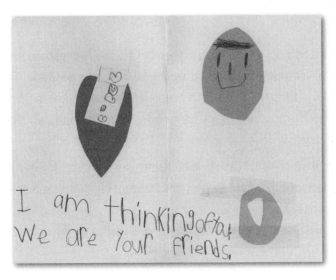

A NOTE TO ANDREW AND CAROLYN FROM THEIR GRADE 1 CLASS.

*

I remember babysitting Sarah before the twins were born and reading her a bedtime story. She told me that I wasn't reading *The Hobbit* right, and she went and retrieved another book, which she presumed I would be able to read. I asked Alan when he returned home what I had missed in the story and he laughed and explained that his version of *The Hobbit* was a bit different from what was printed in the pages of the book.

*

We spent a very contemplative evening last night, playing slow music on the piano and reflecting on life and Alan. We are so very impressed by the great dignity and fortitude with which Alan and you faced this terrible disease. We were privileged to have known Alan and to have shared with him that strong love of nature and the outdoors. It was really good of you, Moyra, to let him have those weekend canoe trips when you had to stay home with the little ones; Alan greatly appreciated this and realized that it was a significant sacrifice for you. Those trips contributed to the good memories that helped to sustain him over these last difficult years. In at least some ways, Alan was a very lucky guy. He had you and three gorgeous children. May you have continued strength and many warm memories.

*

I couldn't help but let you know how sorry I am that Alan passed away. At times, life seems very unfair, ridiculously so. He was a good egg. Too smart by half, I suspect, but that from a moron. I always loved to hear him articulate a perspective or position – always his own, always passionately defended. I feel fortunate to have known him, even for such a short while.

When I think of Alan, I can't help but remember him in kilt. My mum has a couple of favourite "Scottish" expressions that seem somehow appropriate.
"We fear nay foe."
"A coward dies a thousand deaths. The courageous die but once."

*

I really hate this disease. The two of you, though, rose above much of what it can deliver and, in many ways, were victorious. My heartfelt condolences. — (From Dr. P., an oncologist in Toronto whom we had seen early on)

*

I am so glad that I got in to see Alan on Saturday before he died. He looked a lot sicker than he did the last time we met but, amazingly, he was still the same old Alan when we spoke – still cynical about religion, still with at least one joke to tell me. I will miss our chats. We talked on Saturday about Alan's concept of life after death. Alan, as always, could not conceptualize anything other than a void. We then traded jokes and stories and Alan told me that if he had a choice of what animal he could be, he would be a hawk or an eagle. He suggested that this was because he liked to be up high and look down on others with an air of condescension. Of course, this is the way Alan saw himself – an intellectual snob. I suggested to him that he reframe his image of himself – the eagle – to see it as Alan the protector who needed to watch over his children from afar, even after he could no longer be with them in person. He liked this image and expanded on it to say that as an eagle he was too big for the children to capture and bring into the house. I agreed and said that perhaps instead the children would run outside with excitement and point up to the sky and say to each other, "Look up there! There's an eagle." He agreed and we left the discussion of life after death at that. I like to think that Alan is flying around up there now, squawking and shrieking and watching to make sure everything is done correctly. You have had a hard taskmaster to answer to all these months, Moyra. Your job is almost done. — (From Dr. L., Alan's therapist)

I was again comforted by the reference to an eagle. Eagles, hawks, falcons and owls were Alan's favourite creatures, and it was no surprise to me that he chose the image of an untameable bird high in the sky. At my request, my childhood friend Linda created the cover for the order of service for his memorial service. Her eagles were perfect for Alan's last flight.

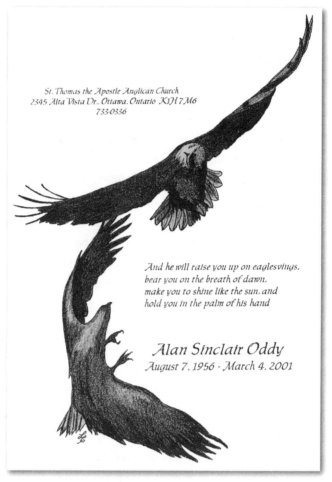

St. Thomas the Apostle Anglican Church
2345 Alta Vista Dr., Ottawa, Ontario K1H 7M6
733-0336

And he will raise you up on eaglesvings,
bear you on the breath of dawn,
make you to shine like the sun, and
hold you in the palm of his hand

Alan Sinclair Oddy
August 7, 1956 - March 4, 2001

By Michael Joncas © 1979, OCP Publications, 5536 NE Hassalo, Portland OR 97213.
All rights reserved. Used with permission.

Monday, March 5, 2001

I am so very comforted by all of your messages. Thank you. I thought you might like to know that the low-toxicity chemo that Alan was on was still working until he died. The tumour was no bigger than it was two months ago. However, his lack of movement contributed to poor circulation. Even though he was checked for clots a week ago, one somehow formed in one leg and then moved into his lungs.

Judging by the speed of his death, the doctors now feel the clot must have been a deep vein thrombosis – from which leg and how remain a mystery. Perhaps it was God's grace that allowed him to avoid the long death by a thousands cuts (Alan's words, not mine). He was aware of us until at least 8:00 a.m. Sunday because he squeezed my hand as I left to go home after spending much of the night with him.

The service is on Saturday at 2:00 p.m. His special causes are the Owl Foundation, the Nature Conservancy of Canada, the Brain Tumour Foundation, the Hospice at May Court and, more lately, Élisabeth Bruyère Health Service (SCO Foundation). There will not be a pre-funeral visitation but there will be a reception after the service.

Alan's corneas were in Toronto by 10:00 this morning. The long bones and heart valves could not be used, since the protocol for steroid users has changed.

Moyra

Wednesday, March 7, 2001 – to Dr. L.

I remember you saying you would stay with us for the journey. I am so glad you saw Alan on Saturday. He was very fond of you. He regarded you as a person of intelligence, and from Alan that is very high praise. It is amazing to me that you were there at the beginning of his illness and by some power I don't pretend to understand you were there at the end.

He was a difficult man to love. I don't understand why or how I continued to love him, but I did and do and always will. I guess it was his angels not his devils that I loved: his wicked sense of humour, his tender love, his keen intelligence (even though he could not remember birthdays). I will always remember, too, the day I stopped wanting him to get better for me and suddenly realized I wanted him to get better for himself. Another phase of growing up even at 42!

I told you several years ago that I wanted the grieving done by the time it happened. I didn't quite make it. No doubt that is healthy, too, in some way.

I knew about Al's love of birds such as eagles and hawks. You will notice the symbolism at the service in several ways. I will tell the children and his parents what he said. They will like it, too.

Your support has meant a great deal to us. You must always remember what a gift you have for healing.

Moyra

Wednesday, March 7, 2001 – to office colleagues

I will send a card later but I wanted to thank all of you for the fruit basket, your support over the last few years, and the memories of Alan that you have shared with me in the last day or so. Through good and bad, Alan and I always had the first-year labs right through to the Ph.D. defences to laugh and cry over.

We are all enjoying the fruit, but Pookie the dog is the most impressed. He thinks the seedless grapes are fantastic fun, and all of us laugh at his antics as he chases them around the house, under beds, behind doors and into small corners. Once he has finished one he runs to the table and woofs for another.

Moyra

Thursday, March 8, 2001 – to a friend

Yesterday I watched Alan's rough-hewn pine box (nothing fancy, at his request) enter the cremation furnace. I thought it would be very hard, but I couldn't help but think Alan would have loved the big burst of flame and the huge woof it made as it came on. By comparison, it was much harder to formally identify him at the funeral home on Tuesday. I went by myself, as Alan had wanted. What a mixture of feelings: intense love, frustration, anger, emptiness, anguish and horrible loneliness. I had him wrapped in a fuzzy flannel sheet with winter teddy bears on it. It was the last sheet set he used at home; he took the pillowslip to the hospital with him.

I keep finding the strength to do the things that need to be done; still, there are lots of tears. I never thought it would be so hard to explain to the children about cremation, for example.

Moyra

Alan had a very simple Committal to Fire service at the crematorium. It seemed I ought to do something more than just send him off all alone, so Fr. Jim offered this service as a possibility. Alan's parents and several other members of his family were there for support. I had not intended that Alan's ashes be at his memorial service on Saturday, but Carolyn was adamant about it, so they were. For the long term, Alan had said he might like his ashes to be placed by the bench near the water at our lake so he can watch the children swim.

For his service, we had a bit of a hunt for hymns that were true to how Alan felt: his love of family, his love of nature, his love of water and of sailing. There were readings, of course, by his brother-in-law Bruce, his close friend Peter and my cousin Marguerite but the one thing Alan had always enjoyed about church was the music. We once attended Evensong at King's College, Cambridge and Alan said it was so beautiful it was almost enough to make even him believe in God. The first hymn, "I Feel the Winds of God" (Jesse Adams, 1908) was perfect for a man who loved to sail. "Today my sail I lift, though heavy oft with drenching spray and torn with many a rift… and brave another cruise." His family hymn, used for several generations, "Unto the Hills" (Marquis of Lorne, 1877), was a given. It begins, "Unto the hills around do I lift up / My longing eyes." We then moved to "For the Beauty of the Earth" (F. S. Pierpoint, 1864), which makes reference to the glory of the skies, hill and vale, tree and flower, sun and moon and stars of night, and the family of brother, sister, parent, child. The final hymn was "The Day Thou Gavest" (Rev. Jon Ellerton, 1870), which includes the line "As o'er each continent and island, the dawn leads on another day."

Long before, Alan had chosen a song for his memorial service. It was Joe Cocker's "Up Where We Belong," from the movie *An Officer and a Gentleman*. It includes the lines "Love lifts us up where we belong, where the eagles cry on a mountain high." The eagle vision was clearly a comfortable one for Alan. More than once in our marriage, we careened down some back road while Alan, at the wheel, tried to see some far off bird of prey, usually a hawk.

Knowing his love of sailing, I had shown Alan the seaman's version of the 23rd psalm some months earlier and he thought he might like it read at his service. He did not know, though, that it would be Sarah who read it. It was her last gift to him – her way of saying goodbye. She was also wearing the ring Alan gave her two years before. He wanted to be the first man to give her a ring. She put it on the day after he died.

> The Lord is my Pilot. I shall not drift. He lighteth me across the dark waters; He steereth me in the deep channels; He keepeth my log. He guideth me by the star of holiness for His name's sake. Yea though I sail amidst the thunders and the tempests of life, I shall dread no danger, for Thou art with me. Thy love and Thy care, they shelter me. Thou preparest a harbour before me in the homeland of eternity; Thou anointest the waves with oil; my ship rideth calmly. Surely sunlight and starlight shall favour me on the voyage I take, and I will rest in the port of my God forever.

Pastor Frank gave the sermon. It seemed right that the two members of the clergy who had ministered to Alan were both involved in his memorial service. The younger children still attend Friendship Club at the church next door, and we think of Pastor Frank as a friend. I think he captured the essence of Alan in his words. The eagles surface again here – partly at my request, because by then I knew of his discussions with Dr. L. the day before he died. Also, I thought the children would like the image – certainly I did – of Daddy as a hawk or untameable eagle, high in the sky.

For Alan Oddy
by Pastor Frank

If I recall correctly, within the first few breaths of our introduction, Al Oddy informed me in no uncertain terms that he had no use for me, the church or God ... though not necessarily in that order. He warned me that he was a heathen, a pagan, and that he liked it that way and had no plans on changing. He may even have wondered if there was a conspiracy afoot to convert him – an impossible task, in his words.

At the end of the evening, he invited me for another visit (or did I invite myself?), provided, of course, that I realized that he was a lost cause. We laughed … and sometime later I did return for another visit, with just him that time – no children to interrupt – though I think Moyra may have hung around in the background (whether to protect him from me or me from him I still don't know). At the end of that afternoon, I took my leave and he informed me that I was welcome any time – provided, of course, that I realized that he was a lost cause, a heathen not about to change.

I'm not sure when it was that we became equals, when he no longer feared that I was visiting just to convert him (or as he mockingly said, *"save his unsaveable soul"*) and when I no longer talked at him or tried to defend my beliefs (for he always had his list of questions ready for my arrival, and in fact e-mailed me at times to warn me of what was coming!). I do know that one day as we talked we just talked – about his feelings of mortality, about his anger and his frustration with the disease, with what it had done to him, with the limitations he felt because of it, even though he was young enough that he should have had no boundaries. We talked about his acceptance – resignation is perhaps a better word – of the course the disease was taking. We talked of his feelings of failure of not being able to control his anger towards those he loved most and of the thought that he had lost his ability to laugh. We talked of his sadness about not being able to see his children grow, of not being able to play with them. We talked of his disappointment that the children saw him as they did – less than strong, less than able, less than perfect.

He hated the fact that he could not finish projects he had started. He despaired that his body let him down, that his energy flagged so easily. After all, *he* was *Alan Oddy*, the man who loved the outdoors, who would be out in a canoe if at all possible (a man who gave me his maps so that *I* could – would – *get out there*).

During those visits we laughed together, we sighed together, we talked with (not at) one another, and we challenged one another to make the most of the time we had left on this earth, to look beyond circumstance and make the most of life, to see not what we didn't get but rather to see what we have.

Alan … Alan had Moyra, with whom he spent half of his life. Alan had his children, who began their invasion of his life eleven years after his marriage. He had family, he had friends, he had hopes. And while he questioned the existence of God he seemed to have an openness (with me, at least) to the possibility of *something else*. So I think that what Jesus said applies to Al and to his struggles. I read again from the Gospel of Matthew and the words of Jesus. We might even personalize these thoughts and title them *Jesus' Invitation to Alan Oddy* (with apologies to Al, who would hate the attention he is getting and the fact that spiritual thoughts might be dedicated to him).

The words of Jesus: *Come to me, all you who labour and are heavy laden, and I will give you rest. Take my yoke upon you and learn from me, for I am gentle and lowly in heart, and you will find rest for your souls. For my yoke is easy and my burden is light* (Matthew 11:28-30).

Jesus' invitation is an invitation to lean. *Come to me, all you who labour and are heavy laden, and I will give you rest.* In other words, *Alan, lean on me.* That was something that Alan had difficulty with. He was *a man.* He was *independent.* He was *strong* – at least until that day after his 20th anniversary when he fell and that hidden weakness was discovered. Yet, as the days and the years passed, Al refused to be anything but strong. He cursed the fact that he might be weak.

He was discouraged that he needed help from anyone (which might be the reason he questioned God so much – why did he need God when he had himself?). He *loathed* being dependent. He didn't seem to want to lean on anyone, but that is God's call to everyone – *lean on me.*

OK, Al was stubborn. Then again, his stubbornness kept him going far longer than anyone expected.

OK, Al was stubborn, but he was learning that he didn't have to be strong all the time. Among other things, he learned that it might be better to walk the hallway with help rather than fall, reinjure himself and be immobile in bed.

That's the next thing we are encouraged to do; Jesus' invitation is an invitation to learn. *Take my yoke upon you and learn from me, for I am gentle and lowly in heart, and you will find rest for your souls.*

Learning involves an open mind, and Al the self-proclaimed agnostic had one. While we may have disagreed on many things religious he was open to continuing the discussions. He was unsure of the existence of God, unsure of the spiritual side of life, but he was still willing to talk about it. In fact, he kept me on my toes with his questions and comments, and though he may not have realized it, helped me to strengthen *my* beliefs!

Perhaps the biggest problem he had with the whole idea of Christianity was that it is so easy. I suggest that Jesus' invitation is an invitation to lightness. *My yoke is easy and my burden is light.* Easy. Al and I talked about God's grace and we talked about God's judgment. We talked about how some people tend to look at God as the law-giving Omnipotent being, who almost delights in condemning people to the fires of hell, and about how the God of the New Testament is the One who reaches out to those who have no hope in anything. We compared the God who threw thunderbolts at sinners with the God who loved people as a gentle shepherd. Alan decided that if there was, indeed, a God, he liked the, uh, *nice* God better.

The *nice* God has a place for his people. Jesus said *In my Father's house are many mansions; if it were not so I would have told you.* The *nice* God has a heaven. The conventional idea of heaven is a place "up there," where angels play harps and people walk on streets of gold.

Alan's heaven is more a place of release. Isaiah says that *those who wait on [God] shall renew their strength; they shall mount up with wings like eagles, they shall run and not be weary, they shall walk and not faint* (Isaiah 40:31). Al might suggest that if he had eagles' wings he could fly above and look down on us with disdain, or he could look down on his family to watch over them and protect them.

Alan's heaven is more a place of freedom, a place with green grass and a sandy beach to build sandcastles on and a stream becoming a river to canoe on, the river running through a wilderness to enjoy, wind rustling through the trees, clean air to breathe, a yell of excitement and exhilaration on his lips.

Alan's heaven is a place of wholeness, a place where people are strong, a place where disease has no hold, a place described by John: *God will wipe away every tear . . . ; there shall be no more death, nor sorrow, nor crying; and there shall be no more pain, for the former things have passed away.*

One evening I happened upon a neighbourhood family. I wish I had met that family earlier. I wish I had met *Al* earlier. He was a good man. A good husband. A good father. A good friend.

Goodbye, Al. Be free.

We closed the service with a Scottish piper's lament, a perfect ending for a man who loved to wear his Cameron kilt. Just before we started our doctorates, we had travelled to Scotland and visited areas of our respective Scottish ancestry. When Alan expressed an interest in having a kilt, I arranged to have one made in the Cameron of Lochiel hunting tartan at the very shop we had visited in Edinburgh. I cannot explain, even now, the cultural pull to that part of our common heritage, but when I hear Celtic music there is a kind of reverberation in my heart. Alan had the same experience.

For some of the congregation, the lament was a trigger for tears. Many remarked afterward that they had been able to hold it together until the lament started on the pipes.

Monday, March 12, 2001

You have all been a source of strength over the last two years. In a way I will miss our regular communication. Thank you to so many of you who wrote, sent cards and flowers and made donations to Al's causes. I will reply to each of you over the course of the next few weeks. Thank you, too, to those of you who came to his service and stayed afterward to share a memory or a hug. It meant so much to all his family.

Afterward, Alan's urn was in the car with us. As I was shouting, "Don't drop Daddy!" Andrew picked it up and commented that Daddy was "still pretty heavy." After we got home, I left the urn out in the living room while I carried in the flowers and cards. I found Andrew snuggled up beside it because, as he put it, "Daddy was cold after being in the car." Children are remarkable at times.

Pookie the dog provided much-needed comic relief throughout all of this by escaping out the door when flowers arrived and heading for the hills with his ears back and his tail straight out, or barking furiously from his perch on a nearby snowbank as fruit baskets arrived. He now figures that he ought to have a bath after the kids. On several nights he has jumped into the tub and waded around in the water after the kids were out. What a strange animal. He and the bird are still friends but a few days ago when he was licking Smokey's back I had to wonder whether it was friendship or tasting.

The children are doing well. They were very tired of the illness and the stress that went with it, and last week they slept a lot. I suppose it's nature's way of healing the hurt and it comes more easily to children than to silly adults.

As a family, the kids and I are doing well, I think. We have ups and downs, but the children are getting lots of mummy time; time that was in short supply while Al was in hospital. We have our moments, though. For example, one day I found a pair of pliers in the wrong place. The kids found me in a puddle shortly after that. Perhaps it was too early, but I gave most of his clothes to the Union Mission. It's a good thing tears help healing.

I am still not sleeping very well, but that is also part of the healing process. I have dreams about Alan, of course: some good, some difficult. I am troubled by the effort he had to make to breathe in his last 24 hours. I will never forget the physical effort it took to take a breath, nor will I forget the last kiss I gave him, at the funeral home.

Mostly, I have a sense of a huge emptiness that used to be fullness. It is this feeling that makes me want to stick my head back under the covers and just sleep – a normal enough reaction, I'm told. Fortunately, the kids, dog and bird prevent me from feeling too sorry for myself. The dog will be "fixed" next week, which should end the awkward explanations that accompany his attempts to mate with every teddy bear in the house! Smokey continues to court the dog. It is quite a sight to see a bird, with wings slightly out, sing a love song to a pup that is so excited by the bird that it is nearly wetting itself. Smokey also spends a lot of time with Carolyn, including sleeping on her shoulder for a good chunk of the night. This means that this morning, for example, I woke up to find Andrew snuggled in on one side of me and Carolyn on the other. The dog was sleeping half on my legs and the bird was settled on Carolyn's back. Sarah, bless her heart, stayed in her own bed. Once everyone was up, the dog upchucked twice on the carpet, which upset Carolyn, who then followed suit. So, as you see, we have a busy life!

The pets are probably the best medicine going. The dog figures, like all dogs do, that he is human. This is why he doesn't eat dog food. He is partial to things like green pepper and frozen raspberries. His favourite main course is roast beef with gravy (no potatoes, though). The bird follows the family around the house, so when I make dinner he is in the kitchen. When the children watch cartoons, he stays with them. He is fond of cuddles and loves it when the kids scratch his cheek patches. One of my girlfriends wondered (to herself) why all the pictures in the house were hanging crooked, until she saw the bird landing on them and bumping them out of position. Hence, there is a sense of everything being a bit out of kilter when you enter the house. It drives neat freaks mad! There was a time when I would have been part of that group, but I have grown beyond that.

The kids and I have received so much comfort from e-mails, cards, letters, flowers and gifts of food. It has been a wonderful support. I continue to fill out life insurance forms. Each one has its own crazy rules. I had to track down the attending physician for signatures and the family physician for more signatures. Papers must be submitted in various combinations of originals, certified copies, double, triple, and of course there is still income tax to do.

Moyra

From Alan

Some days after Alan died, I found the courage to open the envelope he left for me. He had written the letter when he felt strong enough to do so, as he approached the second resection. He had modified it several times, including the previous November, just four months before his death. The letter contains a reference to The House at Pooh Corner. He had loved the story as a child and wanted to leave a legacy of bedtime stories for his own children and so recorded himself reading the entire book for them to listen to.

In his letter to me, it is clear that Alan had also sensed the closing of a door and the knowledge that I would be going on without him. It was not so much Alan's death or his funeral that marked the click of the closing door for me, but reading his final message.

To Moyra, the most important person in my life.

If you are reading this, it means that I have lost my fight and you are now feeling very much alone. It seems like all too few years that we have had together, even if it has been 20 years. We started a wonderful family together. I am so sorry that I'll miss watching the children grow up. They are already children to be proud of. I've left you with a terrible burden; again, all I can say is sorry. This is not how I planned things.

I have left some letters to our guys in my desk. Look in the middle drawer, next to the envelope box and the divider. You can decide when they are ready for them.

I can't find the words to tell you how important you are to me. There has never been anything that ever came close to how important you are to me. I know most of our time together has been spent with you trying to keep me happy. You have taken care of me when I was ill, tolerated me when I was obnoxious, and borne the burden of my depression. That, I would say, pretty much summarises our relationship together. During the seizures, it was a comfort to have you hold my head and talk to me. I have never really understood why you have been so good to me. This early widow-hood is the final insult in a longstanding bad deal for you. I hope you can find someone to share your life with – someone more deserving of your attention, someone who can take care of you, as you ought to be.

Please believe I've done all I could to survive. I wish there had been more. It's too late now in any case. One hope I have is that your career is well enough established that any disruption doesn't cause many consequences.

I can't say that I have any regrets about things I haven't done in my life, apart from learning to ski. It would have been useful in Sweden. If I had any last requests it would be to get a few skiing lessons for Sarah, Andrew and Carolyn, including all the other stuff that will keep you busy. They'll probably all need lessons in self-defence when they are a bit older.

I have even run the spelling checker on this. There, I thought you would be impressed.

This is actually the dedication on The House at Pooh Corner. Although modified a bit, the words are still useful. It applies equally well to our children – when they are behaving themselves.

You gave me Christopher Robin, and then
You breathed new life into Pooh.
Whatever of each has left my pen
Goes homing back to you.

My memories are ready and come to greet
The wife they long to see ——
They would be my present to you, my sweet,
If they weren't your gift to me.

Alan

7

WHEN THE DOOR CLOSES – THE FIRST YEAR

In the first few weeks after Alan's death, there was a feeling of release in my little family. The children slept long hours, as Mother Nature gave them the rest they needed. We focused on the things that needed to be done, such as planning Andrew and Carolyn's seventh birthday party (their first without Alan) and taking care of Pookie the dog. Although I had been told long before that a pet could be an integral part of dealing with grief, I was amazed at how true this was. Pookie would often be found curled up in someone's arms, in a lap or in a bed. He received, and gave, unconditional love at the time when we all needed it most.

As Alan's illness unfolded, I had understood all too well that I would be going on without him. However, as the door slowly closed, I became more confident in myself. I emerged, after Alan's death, knowing that I had the ability to care for the kids and hold on to a career. I followed the age-old advice to make no major decisions in that first year. It made good sense to stay where I was, in the life that we had, supported by the same group of family and friends. Still, the upheaval and change were significant. Decisions had to be made about the family and how to cope, and, of course, the estate issues had to be handled. In the grand scheme of things, and when compared to poverty, floods and hurricanes, these were small issues, but they felt very big at times. Still, they were issues that had to be faced and they dominated life for a while, since the need to secure the family's future was a priority.

Early in Alan's illness, we had sought the advice of a financial adviser and implemented a plan that would not need to be changed for some time. I was fortunate to be able carry on as I had been doing. I was able to keep our home, the after-school child care arrangements were in place, and my career was established and stable. Still, I could not think, in those early days, of building that career. I focused simply on moving forward.

Alan's cousin Janet and I kept in touch and were glad to hear each other's news.

Tuesday, April 3, 2001 – from Janet, referring to her brain tumour support group

Last night, I went to my first support group meeting since Alan died. I just had to take a break and go on a little denial vacation for a couple of weeks. The news of his death hit me harder than I expected. The hardest part was telling my friend who is currently in a nursing home (180 miles away from here) that Alan had died. I read him your letter about the blood clot being the culprit, not the tumour. I think that encouraged him. People don't have any idea how to deal with people with brain tumours. It used to make me feel like I was contagious. Enough bitching. Sorry.

Janet

Meanwhile, I continued to write to my own support group of family, friends and colleagues.

Monday, April 9, 2001

Grumble, grumble.

Due to birthday parties (one of the guests had stomach flu and upchucked all over the tumble track at the gymnastics centre; another thought my idea of a ball, a hula hoop and a skipping rope as loot was dumb) and complications from neutering poor old Pookie (whose bottom is now swollen to several times the size of the offending wee scrotum and who cost me $$$ in ER at the animal hospital late last night), my grand plans to complete my marking were scuttled.

Hence, I will stay home and attempt to recover the marking time, in the comfort of my home office. I just love kids and dogs and husbands. Whatever would I do on my weekends without such excitement to keep me busy?

Thank you, God, for giving me a sense of humour!

Moyra

Monday, April 16, 2001 – to a friend

I will likely need company at some point. I am still marking. There is no time to feel very sorry for myself (yet). I am waiting for the big crash. Easter was a good challenge. I did the church thing and was okay there. I had thought the emotional memory would be too hard. Dinner was harder. It was the first big feast without Alan since I was nineteen or 20.

I am taking the kids to Florida for a week in early May for a bit of R&R. We will meet some friends and their kids there, so it will be quite an adventure. I was of two minds on this one, because I had sort of promised Alan we would travel again someday when he was able to. He had wanted to go to the beach one more time. It feels wrong to do it without him, and yet we are without him.

I am told this is a good thing to do after a long, hard winter – both for them and for me. I even bought a new bathing suit with a built-in push-up bra. I giggled over that for half an hour.

Moyra

Saturday, April 21, 2001

Last night, when we were all snuggled in bed, Andrew brought me the monkey I got Al to hug in the hospital – the nurses called it Little Buddy. Andrew told me that Buddy needed to sleep with me because he was really sad that Daddy had died. So I hugged Buddy, and Andrew hugged Buddy, and I hugged Andrew. Then I checked my information on children and grief.

In my reading (do you suppose people trained in research ever stop researching?) of *Caregiving: The Spiritual Journey of Love, Loss and Renewal*, I recognize myself in the appropriate sections. It's a little disconcerting to read about yourself and realize it applies to so many people, and not just in death. I am working through the renewal section. (My other bedtime reading is *Facing a Death in the Family: A Legal and Practical Guide*.)

Our trip to Florida will be squished into the available space between my job stuff and Sarah's choir commitments. A family member will be Pookie-, Smokey-, fish- and house-sitting. It will be interesting for him to look after a small dog and an insane bird, rather than the big beasts he lives with normally.

Moyra

Thursday, May 24, 2001

We are doing all right, I think – not normal yet, but not too bad. Andrew spends a lot of time at night hugging the little monkey that Alan kept in his hospital bed, and has expressed worry that his son might get brain cancer. Carolyn is apparently very nurturing at school. I guess she is replacing visiting her dad daily with sitting at lunch with one of the disabled kids at school. She still finds comfort in sleeping in Al's bed at home. Sarah seems to be doing the best for now. All the anger she had at her dad for being sick has gone. She seems to find it comforting to wear the ring he gave her two years ago. We can even joke about the traits she shares with her dad, including gluttony for chips at family gatherings.

I am, I suppose, running about a C grade, which is satisfactory. I am busy, and am enjoying that part. I get thrown by things at odd times, though.

We went to the lake on the weekend and Al's trapeze for pulling himself up in our bed was there waiting for him, and his lake shoes were sitting in their usual spot by the bed. All of his really special lake things were out – I had forgotten that I had left them out on our last visit when we closed up the cabin. Fortunately, Pookie was there to take my mind off things. He thinks the lake is doggy paradise and ran back and forth from the cabin to the water and back over and over again. He enjoyed following Andrew into the bushy part of our property where Carolyn, Andrew and a friend were building a fort. When the sun went down, Pookie snuggled on the bed with Sarah and her friend, squishing himself between them and charming them with his wet-nose-in-the-face routine early the next morning.

The early mornings are the worst time for me. The old bit about the day being coldest and darkest just before dawn is true in more ways than one. Then, of course, the dog sticks his cold, wet nose in my face to tell me he needs to go out, and then the kids need breakfast, and the fights break out over toast, and the day begins, and I have no time to feel sorry for myself.

The trip to Florida was a success. We went to Orlando, a place Alan would not have chosen to go (no beach). Of course, we had to do the Disney thing: Animal Kingdom, Magic Kingdom and EPCOT. The kids had a great time with our friends. The trip was part of establishing a new family identity. I think I did most of that part; the kids just had a blast.

I am still trying to reassess what I want/need to do in the next months and years. The fun seems to have gone out of the research game for me, although I continue to plod along. Somehow, the importance of "publish or perish" seems trivial in the larger scheme of things. Still, I will give it some time.

Moyra

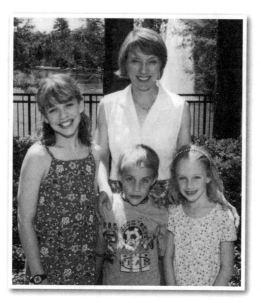

SARAH, ANDREW, MOYRA AND CAROLYN IN ORLANDO.

Saturday, June 16, 2001

Today was one of those days that you wish you could live over again but do differently. Our plans for the day slowly fell apart. We were heading for the lake for Father's Day – Al's favourite place. I was packing the car and Pookie was staying in the house by command as I went in and out. He rarely runs out now if he is under the stay command. Of course, at one point he heard the sound of his archenemy, a car, and he squeezed past my leg and foot in the door, ran down the driveway and under the wheels of a van. Three seconds either way and it would have been different.

He didn't make it to the animal hospital emergency. The vet tried to resuscitate him when I told her that the kids had lost their dad a few months ago. She was very upset. Did you know that vets can swear at least as well as engineers? She waived all the fees and then spent some time brushing him and removing his collar and wrapping him up in a towel so that the kids could stroke him at home.

It broke the kids' hearts when I told them, although Carolyn who had seen the incident, was expecting a bad outcome. The driver didn't stand a chance with a dog that small; a big black lab would have caught her eye. I remember that he ran straight back to me, but there was little I could do except wrap him up and keep him calm. Then the children ran to me to have me make it all better, too. Kisses just can't fix that kind of injury – to the dog or the kids. Mums just can't make it all better.

The dog was part of why we are doing as well as we are – demanding attention and lavishing love and generally being a schnook, stealing the kids' toys and challenging them to catch him. We will have to get another pup when the time is right. Perhaps this time we'll get a regular shoe-eating variety, rather than a car-chasing variety. He has been such a good thing for us as a family, and even the few times he spent with Alan were very special for Alan. Pookie seemed to agree with Alan that hospital shepherd's pie was the best.

Moyra

The children's book *Water Bugs and Dragonflies* by Doris Stickney (United Church Press) explains death in terms that a child can understand. My children found it very comforting when their dad died, and when Pookie died, we read it again. It is the simple, very sweet story of a group of water bugs that watch other water bugs climb a stalk and disappear above the water. They all promise that when their turn comes, they will come back and tell the others what is above the water's surface. When the first of the friends climbs the stalk and turns into a dragonfly, it finds it cannot go back into the pond to tell the other bugs how wonderful it is. The dragonfly, knowing its friends will understand in time, flies off to its new life.

Sunday, June 17, 2001

As you might have guessed, we had a long night of "Why does everything I love die?" In the words of one of you, the timing really sucks. This morning, on Father's Day no less, when the sobbing started up again, we discussed the idea of another puppy in a few weeks or months and Sarah said, "I need something to love right now." Clearly, the little fellow was a big part of helping them get over Al's long illness. Andrew thought a cat would be fine, as he had wanted to stroke something soft. Carolyn said a rabbit would be good, as she could carry it around.

The adoption centre at the Humane Society was closed, so I said we could go look at the pet store where Pookie came from. I figured I was in for a guinea pig, perhaps, or another bird at the worst – something small but cuddly and a cage or two. HA!

We are now the proud, but poorer, owners of a four-month-old Pomeranian pup that shares a few physical characteristics with Pookie. I sent the kids into the dog play area at the store with the pup and he adopted them on the spot, covered them with kisses and they all fell in love. Does it help that the dog was on sale because he was older than most?

They are still very sad about Pookie and tears are shed from time to time, but there is a soft, fluffy fellow all ready now to hold when the tears come. So now we are back to puddles on the floor and neutering and worming and getting up in the night and a little warm body for them to hug when they feel lonely. His name is Scooter (or Scootie).

Moyra

There were times when I simply followed my instincts, and this was one of them. My head said to wait awhile before getting another dog, but my heart, my inner instinct – the same one I had responded to when I purchased Pookie – told me to give the children something to love as quickly as I could. They were grieving for their dad and now also the little creature that somehow helped them deal with the loss of their dad. It just felt right and we never looked back. Scooter immediately became a full member of the family. It wasn't until a few months later that we learned that the folks at the pet store referred to him as "that insane Pomeranian." They were right!

Monday, July 23, 2001

All's well here. We just had a week at the lake. It was lovely, although the missing Alan part was pretty strong for me. I had a couple of those "he'll never see this, walk here, come around that corner again" episodes. When that happens I just want to crawl into bed and go back to sleep.

The cabin is reaching a state of usefulness now; it is more fun and less work. I still need to insulate the sucker, but before I do that, I have to decide about propane versus electricity, so perhaps I can avoid the issue for another season or two.

I painted the floor again, and now it is a mix of big yellow, white and grey squares matching the size of the 4x4, 4x8 or 2x8 sheets of plywood. It looks neat. The part we especially like are the little doggy prints; some are Pookie's. More recently, Scootie added his set. There are matching prints on the deck outside where little paws were put after they got into the cabin for a quick walkabout. The kids want me to leave the prints. Sarah thinks it adds character. Maybe next week we'll add a set of human handprints and footprints, and that will make it look deliberate.

The dock is in deep water this year, after several years in shallow water for kid safety. This has improved swimming greatly. Andrew now swims under the dock with his mask looking at fish! Sarah is much happier without the threat of a bit of green stuff wrapping itself around her leg and sucking her to the bottom of the bog. Carolyn is a bit of a fish, so she is pleased, too. The paddleboat has been a real addition and they have a great time in it, too. A few days ago, Sarah and Andrew were out and Sarah was freaking out about a giant dock spider in the boat. Normally, Sarah is the big sister, calm and in control. I had to call to Andrew to rescue his sister by picking up the spider and tossing it over the side. Andrew was happy to pick it up but didn't like the idea of tossing it. Finally, he was convinced. It turned out it was a water walker-hopper, because it just stood up and walked-hopped to shore. Later on, Andrew found a nice big snake and was busy stroking its tail when I arrived.

Moyra

This very long snake turned out to be a Black Rat snake. A little research revealed that in our area the Black Rat snake is a threatened species. We still keep a watch out for them at the lake. These arboreal snakes can surprise one by hanging off a tree branch. Mostly, though, we see them sunning on a rock or slowly moving from one part of the property to another.

Tuesday, July 24, 2001 – to a colleague overseas

I've known you are out there and thinking of us. I think each person has dealt with Al's illness and death in his or her own way. It seems to me that the men are particularly troubled by it. I think we are all bothered most by the fact it was brain cancer. We intellectuals live by our brains, and I think we feel it differently than others. I suppose it might be a bit like a concert pianist losing an arm.

Alan enjoyed his visits to your group. He was fond of your graduate students, too, and I think influenced them more than he would have if he had been on faculty. He liked his solitary work and then occasional bursts into the community. He often wondered whether he should have been on faculty, but he would have hated the administrivia we deal with, and he had little patience with students bugging me, let alone him. I recall him sounding off at one of my students when he felt the question was silly. I had to tell him afterward to stay out of dealing with my people, no matter how stupid they seemed to be.

We are muddling along. I still haven't found my feet and the doctors tell me I shouldn't have unrealistic expectations of returning to the woman I was three years ago. I guess I must accept that I will find a new path at some point and not fight it too much. It seems rather painful to work on our joint code now that Alan is gone, but this should ease with time. So much of us as partners is buried in it, some things going all the way back to our Ph.D.s, starting in 1983! It's also hard to deal with the fact that I've lost my biggest user and tester. What is the point of creating a new element, let's say, just for me? Alan used to take the stuff I did, mix it with the stuff he did and use it in his work for people like you.

Moyra

Tuesday, September 11, 2001

Sarah had already left for school and I was at home, preparing to take Andrew and Carolyn to school when the first plane hit the World Trade Center in New York. I felt again, as I had years earlier in the Emergency Room, the sense of time stopping. I found myself sitting on my bed, crying, not for me and not for my children but for all those families who were suddenly entering a world of upheaval, uncertainty and grief. In the evening I hugged each of my three beautiful children and again, consciously, counted my many blessings.

Moyra

Monday, October 1, 2001

The kids and I went canoe-camping this weekend with ten other people from my office. We had a great time, bruises, bumps and other aches notwithstanding. The dog went with us. He is a great wilderness dog, staying close but having a gas. The birds – yes, birds; we have a lovebird named Sweety to keep Smokey company – stayed home.

We all crammed into the tent Alan bought for his birthday just before his diagnosis. He was really ticked that he never got a chance to use it, so we baptized it with dew and lake water this weekend. It was cold, but with the four of us and the dog inside we stayed warm. Sarah went out to the privy (very rudimentary) at 4:00 a.m. and accidentally left the zipper a bit open. I woke up a while later and did a head count and came up one furry head short. Scootie was having a wonderful time outside in the moonlight. He came in when called – fortunately – and promptly dug his way into my sleeping bag.

The kids were wonderful, apart from a variety of squabbles between Andrew and Carolyn in particular. Sarah is a pretty good bow paddler now. We remembered Alan and me when I was a stern paddler. Alan, no matter how hard he tried, could not prevent himself from correcting me, and my steering, whenever he was in the bow. Eventually I just told him to stay in the stern, as it made my life easier. We had to laugh when Andrew started to correct my steering when he was in the middle seat! My steering is fine, by the way.

I got up early on Sunday morning and watched the mist rise off the lake for Alan, because that is what he liked to do. All in all, it was exhausting but fun, and Carolyn wants to do it again. Andrew brought home a pocketful of rocks to identify. Sarah was pleased to be second in command, although she had a long cry Saturday night, missing Alan. She can remember the very few trips she went on with the two of us.

Moyra

Tuesday, November 13, 2001

Alan's ashes are happily perched on the bedroom closet shelf, where he can observe all that goes on around here. Why, just last night I heard him muttering about the dog being allowed to sleep on the sheets, the kids being up too late again and Sarah not doing her homework!

I had once promised Alan that the dog would never sleep in the bed. Well, when Scootie was neutered, he dug himself a nice little nest under the covers when none of us was watching. He has since become a regular, waiting until I am in a deep sleep and then sneaking in from the far side until he is on the sheets and often squiggling around until he has his head resting on a nearby pillow. I took a picture of him a few days ago, sleeping next to Andrew. The two of them were sharing the same pillow, with the covers pulled up to their ears, and Scootie had his paw resting on Andrew's open lips.

This is a clever dog. Just this weekend, he extended his skill set to getting over the virtual fence around the yard! He runs full tilt, and then jumps high and over buried fence wire to the sounds of the warning beeps and the spray of citronella. When he lands, he turns back and looks at the fence line and then heads for the hills to torment other dogs walking in the field, rolling in such delights as doggy doo-doo and vocally address-ing the local squirrel population.

I expect to devote some time to trying to adjust the take-off area to prevent further fun. In the meantime, he is tied up again, much to his disgust. Puppy school is helping, but last week we were given the award for most enthusiastic dog. I think that means he is the happiest and least obedient.

I still dream way too much about Alan. The dreams are vivid and are fre-quently the same, so I am able to remember them when I wake up, which is unusual for me. I have to sort out what is real and what is dreaming. One day, I spent a few minutes trying to recall who I was. Then I had to sort out that Alan was my only husband and that the other husband was a dream. I realized that the old brain was trying to put the good years into one file folder and the difficult years of depression and cancer into an-other. Fortunately, the messages are not overly complex in these dreams, so I don't yet need a shrink. I don't mind the happy-healthy dreams but I am coming to dread waking up crying or angry or confused from one of the dreams that relives his diagnosis, illness, treatment and death. I hope they will ease off as time goes by. I assume by then that my brain will have processed and sorted through all the relevant data.

The kids talk about their dad a lot. Sarah was remembering just the other day what she did when she was home sick and Alan was on Daddy duty. She used to sneak into his office and shout "Boo!" at him. Sarah and I also had a chat about one of her teachers and I found myself giving the "maybe she was having a bad day" talk. Then I said to Sarah, "Do you want to know what your dad would say?" When she agreed, I told her that Alan would say, "The woman is a silly old cow." We had a good laugh over that and Sarah felt much better. Andrew and Carolyn have fewer strong memories but often surprise me with what they do recall.

For the most part, I have less trouble keeping a smile on my face after I paste it there in the morning. There is a lot to do, and just doing my job and raising the kids keeps me from feeling too sorry for myself. I have noticed that I am starting to appreciate the various physical attributes of the males of the species. I had forgotten how attractive I used to find broad shoulders and strong hands. I suppose it's a sign of healing, but it's kind of useless at this point. I mean, what good is a sex drive now?

Moyra

Thursday, November 22, 2001

Scooter is a high-energy pup. He loved puppy school and made friends with all the other dogs there. To my amazement, we were given a certificate of completion, even though he was weak on all the elements of the first level, including heel and stay. He was good on the sit and come sequence and he was the only one in the class to successfully retrieve, so we passed the course on bonus marks, I think. I have since learned that Pomeranians score one out of five for trainability. In any case, it became apparent that Scooter needed a buddy especially since he had mastered the art of jumping the virtual fence in several spots and was going to the field to help walk other people's dogs!

At puppy school, Scoot became quite attached to a little female his own size and made eyes at her all the time. She was eight years old and flirted with him outrageously, lifting her leg so he could sniff. He seems to like girl dogs, despite the obvious removal of key parts of his anatomy. I guess the instincts never go away. We began looking about a month ago for the right buddy; we almost took a Sheltie from a breeder who is trying to downsize her home kennel. In the end, we didn't because the dog was six, and I wasn't sure she could keep up with Scooter, although she was a beautiful, sweet-natured lady dog.

Last night, after finally convincing Carolyn that her hair needed cutting, we passed by the pet store and there she was, a miniature schnauzer, 3 pounds and eleven weeks of grey fuzz. We brought her home and she and Scoot were bonded in minutes. She spent much of the evening setting the much bigger Scooter in his place. They played such games as "my bone – your bone," "tug of war" and "tag, you're it." At one point, Scoot was dragging her by the ear down the hall and she was happy as a clam. A few minutes later, she was lying on him chewing his ear.

Her name is Penelope, but we call her Penny. Yours in the insanity of parenthood, because, really, there is no sane reason to have either kids or dogs or cats or birds, but they sure are cute.

Moyra

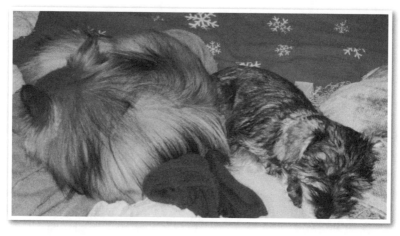

SCOOTER AND TINY PENNY, ASLEEP ON MY PILLOWS, AFTER HUNTING FOR SOCKS.

Wednesday, December 12, 2001

Our first Christmas without Alan is approaching. Today is probably typical of many of our days and just a little too exciting. It began very early, when an alarm went off. In my lovely, all-too-rare deep sleep, I assumed first that it was the television – that hum it makes in the night when programming ends. After the remote control failed to stop the ringing, I assumed it was the carbon monoxide detector and threw open the patio door and began to get the kids up. At about this point, with two dogs, three kids and one of the birds around me, I realized it was the smoke alarm. Still, there was no smoke, so I figured we had a spider in the detector. I began to try to turn off the alarm and the klaxon in the ceiling. (This is trickier than you might think with a monitored alarm with no battery and a spider in the works.) Right then, the alarm company called to tell me they had detected an intruder alarm! I think a big truck had gone through the neighbourhood and disconnected the magnets long enough to send the signal. Sarah managed to deactivate the bells, the kids retreated to bed, and I was left with the dogs and wide-open eyes. Of course, if I had checked the alarm first and seen which zone was screaming, I would have known the alarm was triggered by an external door that had not been shut properly.

Emotionally, we are feeling much better. Once in a while, I feel the old me popping out and am surprised by the good feeling of just being me. I am still dreaming about Alan. I still feel a bit lost career-wise. I can't quite figure out how to do it all and so I have resorted to trying to catch the dropped balls on the first bounce. My goal for the moment is to point in the right direction and see where I end up.

The children, however, seem to be adjusting well, even if I find the number of cookies required at this time of year is excessive for three children in various activities. Sarah is doing very well in school, but, like most parents, I cringe when she approaches me at 9:00 p.m. to announce that xyz is due tomorrow and do you, Mummy, have any information on abc? I can't tell you how pleased I am that she is not allowed to bring her cello home from school. I can just see me trying to explain to the principal how two dogs and a couple of birds nibbled Sarah's instrument. Smokey is still trying to make eggs with Carolyn. Sarah's collection of close friends includes a couple of kids living with just one parent. I think she finds them a help. No doubt they each gripe about their respective aging parent.

Andrew has trouble sometimes with the uncertainly of life but generally focuses on annoying his twin sister. Carolyn still bobs like a cork in the water but also loves to bug Andrew to distraction. To call our home a chaotic zoo would be polite. A friend asked why I don't hire a housekeeper to help out. I replied that it would hardly be worth it; the help would have to come every day.

I wish you all peace and comfort for the year to come. You have continued to support me in the last few months. It has been a lesson in life and friendship.

Moyra

I was ready to let go of my virtual support group, and this update, with its Christmas thank you, was the last e-mail I sent to the group that had meant so much to me throughout Alan's illness and the first part of the healing process. This part of my long record and documentation of Alan's illness was now complete.

We had begun to establish a new family identity that seemed to work. For me, there was comfort to be found in the simple structure and routine of school, work and children's activities. It became easier as the months passed, as did all the major events without Alan: the children's birthdays, holidays on our own, his birthday, our anniversary, Thanksgiving, my birthday, and now Alan's favourite, Christmas.

On Christmas morning, I looked at my children and took this picture. Andrew, a young man with scientific interests in such things as artillery, wearing his choice of mismatched pyjamas is on the right, actively teasing Carolyn. Carolyn, my fashion-conscious, piano-playing, Friendship Club attender, and Brownie, is in the middle, holding Scooter. Scooter, who will always believe he is just a small, furry four-legged human, not a Pomeranian, was in mid-chew on Penelope, the miniature Schnauzer, when the flash went off, leaving him embarrassingly open-mouthed.

Sarah holds Penny. Sarah, by then a piano- and cello-playing, singing, braces-wearing math-whiz teenager, was roused from sleep (is it any wonder?) by her younger siblings. Mercifully, the birds were still in their cage and not flying about the house, although they were screeching madly to help us celebrate the significance of the day. You can use your imagination to picture me: I had completed wrapping only a few hours earlier and required a fortified coffee shortly after this family portrait moment.

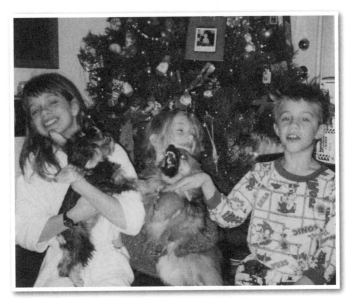

SARAH (HOLDING PENNY), CAROLYN (HOLDING SCOOTER) AND ANDREW ON CHRISTMAS MORNING.

Common wisdom says that the first year following the loss is the worst, and then it gets better. The idea that it will be a year until you feel better is pretty hard to take, especially right after the hard sledding of the diagnosis-to-death phase. I recall being a new mum and being told that colic usually ends by the time the baby is three months old. Three months! It might as well have been a lifetime. The time is still too long; you want the baby to feel better now. The same is true after the death of someone you love: you want to feel better now, and you want your family to feel better now, not after a year. Of course I knew, logically, that it would take time to make the transition. The one-year time frame again gave me a point in time and space at which to aim, and it fit nicely with my one-day-at-a-time approach. I reached the end of the first year expecting to feel, once again, somehow complete, but I didn't feel complete. I was healthy, things were going well, and the children were busy and thriving, but I felt a bit lost. I was only partway there.

Still, the year of not making major decisions had passed and I had to begin to venture into new territory – where decisions had to be made by me alone. The first year had given me the confidence and knowledge to face the second one.

8

2002 – 2005
FINDING A NEW PATH

Who am I?

I continued one day at a time, one foot in front of the other: work, home and kids. I was comfortable with this. It seemed to be working well and things were progressing. Naturally, my focus continued to be on keeping the kids' lives moving forward at school and in their chosen activities, and also on their emotional and physical health. I still relied frequently on friends and family to drive children to various activities at various times but the need was lessening. While I understood my role with respect to the children, I had not yet reached the stage at which I understood what I needed to do for myself to move forward.

My sense of feeling a little lost related, I think, to needing to resolve something about my identity. In the stages of my life so far, I had been first a daughter and a sister, and then a university student, a wife, an employee, a doctoral candidate, a mother and a professor. Now, while I remained a daughter and a sister, for example, I was no longer a wife. I was half a couple. The me of my teens, who had existed before Alan, and who had run full tilt at waist-high fences and had held a number of hurdling records, was gone. I had fallen in love with Alan as a very enthusiastic young woman still in my undergraduate years, and our lives had been entwined ever since. The university student who had charged at new challenges and higher degrees was long gone.

As a wife and later as a mother, I had tried to accommodate the ups and downs that accompanied Alan's struggle with depression. Over time, we had become career research partners. It was a wonderful and productive partnership, albeit fraught with the many challenges of combining my career, his business and our home life. This research relationship was, as far as we knew, unique in our area. Without him, I lost the part of my research enterprise that shepherded my research developments from the halls of academia to use in the outside world. It is a loss from which I was unlikely to ever fully recover, if indeed I even wished to.

Ultimately, I was not the same pony-tailed girl Alan had met in first-year engineering, nor the woman he had worked with, nor the woman who had stood by him throughout his illness. I had to accept that I could not map out a route for my future all at once. I did not know who I was underneath, and had to trust that the person who emerged was someone with whom I could get along. I decided consciously to allow myself the time to establish a new me, based on the simple goal of taking things one day at a time and having the faith that if I walked down the road I would end up in a suitable place. Later, when I read these words by the Rev. Dr. Tom Sherwood of the Ecumenical Chaplaincy at Carleton University, my understanding of how to proceed made even more sense.

> We often think of sacred space as place rather than journey. But usually, faith is the way rather than the destination, and a pilgrimage is a sacred place all along its way.
>
> In our mind's eye, sacred places usually look more like churches and shrines, mosques and temples, mountains and gardens, than escalators or pathways.

But if the journey we undertake living our lives is truly a response to God's call, then every step is an expression of faith, and God is with us every metre, [in] every decision, every task, every course, every project, every setback, every success, every experience, every moment … and each place we step, each pace, is a sacred place.

One of the setbacks we experienced was the loss of Carolyn's bedtime companion, Smokey the cockatiel. After searching the house high and low, we concluded that he had flown out an open door. In due course, Sunny, a yellow lovebird, joined Sweetie and we found out why lovebirds are called lovebirds: they sit, eat and sleep together constantly.

Loneliness was a frequent night-time visitor, especially when family and work chaos was high, but I was more easily able to summon good memories and gentle thoughts for comfort. Still, it was possible to be blindsided by sadness. More than once I was reduced to tears when I found a note tucked in a book or a familiar song played on the radio. "Up Where We Belong," which Alan had chosen for his memorial service, and Louis Armstrong's "What a Wonderful World," which had been popular when we started our doctorates, had the power to trip me up. On one occasion, I found a note Alan had written to me and left in his desk. Among other things, it instructed me to "give Tom the plaque." It took me a long time to realize that he was talking about a brass plaque that he and a childhood friend had liberated from a piece of heavy machinery. Of course, when I realized what it was, I sent it off to Tom, who in turn was deeply moved when the plaque fell out of the padded envelope.

While loneliness visited at night, tiredness was my daytime companion. It was a different kind of tired than I had experienced when Alan was ill. Then I would have described myself as being in a state of chronic exhaustion. This tiredness was more of a worn down, dragging my feet kind of feeling. I tried to be realistic. I was on my own with three young kids, after nearly 25 years of being part of a vital couple.

Still, I promised myself that since the children could now manage on their own for a while, I could go out for coffee or to lunch or dinner from time to time with friends or office colleagues. On one occasion, however, I bravely met an unattached male acquaintance for lunch. At dessert time, my cell phone rang. It was the secretary at Carolyn's school, who told me that Carolyn appeared to have broken her nose and would I please come and retrieve her. (Carolyn had turned around at the end of a race to witness the arrival of the second-place person. His forehead and Carolyn's nose collided.) Lunch was over. So much for a leisurely coffee and chat. That afternoon, Carolyn and I checked with the doctor and received instructions on how to get through the next few days, as her nose healed.

Those few days had passed when we went to the lake. Carolyn was healing nicely and the blue smudges around her eyes were fading, but within hours we were at it again, when she fell off the swing. After the tears had stopped, and the Tylenol had taken effect, all seemed well and there was no bruising or bleeding. The next day, though, it was clear that she was not using her arm properly, although she did not seem to be in pain. Sure enough, X-rays showed she had cracked the bone in her upper arm (the humerus). The break was not in a location amenable to taking a cast, so she was trussed up like a chicken in a sling and ordered to stay quiet for four weeks. (I didn't mention that this would be virtually impossible!) Fortunately, at the end of the first two weeks, the doctor freed her from the sling and cleared her for gentle activity. The bone had not yet healed, of course, but she had a full range of motion and no pain. The swing and other vigorous activities were off limits for another month. Compared to the complete lack of movement that had been initially prescribed, this was a huge relief.

Over the next eight weeks, Scooter was sprayed at close range by a skunk, Penny tangled twice with a porcupine at the lake, and Andrew slipped on a climber, breaking one of his permanent front teeth. It was clear to me that making the rounds of doctors, X-ray technicians, dentists, emergency room staff and very nice, but expensive, country veterinarians was not best way to deal with loneliness.

As I grappled with loneliness, I began to feel that part of the solution was to bring meaning to everything that had happened. Surely there was a greater good that could come out of the collective experiences of the individuals involved? Surely these experiences could contribute to making something better, somehow? I needed to give them shape and meaning and so I continued to add to the logbook, knowing, at the very least, that I would complete the record for the children.

Alan had also felt the need to give meaning to it all and, in his last few months, he had asked that I do something for each of the children's schools. I hadn't done anything about it yet, as I was waiting for a bit of inspiration. Sarah had commented several times that her new school looked like a jail, so I made a donation to cover the cost of paint for the lockers. For Andrew and Carolyn's school, I made a donation towards the purchase of team pinnies for their various sporting competitions, such as cross-country running and track and field.

On a personal level, I began to reposition myself both at home and at work, so that I could begin to make some sort of personally mean-ingful contribution to the bigger picture. Some things were easily implemented: I became a more regular blood donor and I increased my charitable donations. I made a promise to myself to spend a little more time at the children's schools, sometimes to talk about some aspect of engineering, sometimes to help supervise activities. With the very successful conclusion of the 2002 International Conference of Women Engineers and Scientists, which I helped organize, I accepted the role of Associate Chair (Undergraduate) in my department at the university. This is an administrative and service role that includes a good deal of student advising. While time consuming, it's valuable to the students. I continued to enjoy teaching, at both the undergraduate and gradu-ate levels, but I decided I had to be braver about making changes and taking chances. With shaking knees and the permission of the university, I accepted a part-time appointment with the Canadian Nuclear Safety Commission, a quasi-judicial tribunal. This appointment came completely out of the blue, but since the mandate of the Commission is first and foremost that of public safety, the timing, with respect to giving meaning to things, was fortuitous.

Taking the appointment meant I had to further reduce the time available in my life for research. Research builds on the work of others and is generally carried out in small steps. Usually, a step is presented to the research community through a peer-reviewed journal, conference paper or, from time to time, even a book. For me, publishing and presenting the technical work no longer brought the academic thrill and reward it once had. It was the combination of doing the technical research and supporting students in general and women in engineering in particular that had become most rewarding.

In the early years of my career, I had not intended to do any research in the area of women in engineering, a field that was by then opening to women. Still, I had been one of a very few women in my engineering undergraduate class and in my first two jobs in industry. Several years later, I was the first woman to earn a Ph.D. in Mechanical Engineering at Carleton University and the first woman to be appointed as an Assistant Professor in the Faculty of Engineering. Then, in December 1989, fourteen innocent women, most of them engineering students, were murdered at École Polytechnique in Montréal. I felt compelled to honour the memory of all of them in some tangible way. From that time, it was important to me to do research in this area, along with my technical work, even as I became the first woman in engineering at Carleton to progress through the ranks to Associate and then to Full Professor.

I understood that my dual research interests were a little irregular, but they may have contributed to my receiving two honours: the Ottawa

YMCA-YWCA Woman of Distinction Award for Education in 2002, and my 2004 appointment as a Fellow of the Canadian Academy of Engineering. I now acknowledged my difference, my irregularity, perhaps more comfortably than I had done when I began my career in engineering.

About the same time, I realized that my dutifully documented logbook, which I intended to distribute to the family, was becoming more than a family record and legacy for our children, and might have a broader relevance. Perhaps our experience with an aggressive and terminal illness was something that other families could connect with at some level. Perhaps it should be shared, and even published.

Finding the Open Door

As we moved into the third year after Alan's death, I found that I had become, in many ways, a more capable person. Without the other person to share the load, you just make do or adjust. That is not to say I did it all alone. I continued to rely on family and friends, especially for driving Sarah to her activities, since Andrew and Carolyn were too young to be left alone. Alan's mother and Sarah's godparents, Alan's sister Trish and her husband, Bruce, as well as my cousin Marguerite, continued to pitch in faithfully whenever asked. The father of one of Sarah's friends drove Sarah to school nearly every day for a year so she could practise the cello in the music room before class. He drove her to early practice on Friday mornings for another year. A single parent himself, he knew instinctively how to help. How do you thank someone for that kind of gift?

The children became older, more self-reliant and more capable. Each learned to do things they might not have learned had they had both parents. We had to do it, whatever it was, as a family. Things like putting the dock in at the lake became something we did together as a challenge. Each year we have tried to better the time it took the previous year to get the dock either into the water or out of the water.

As the children grow older and stronger, it becomes easier and easier. We even insulated the cabin and put up tongue-and-groove pine on the walls together. Granted, I did the bulk of it, but they were involved. Are they better than they would have been with their dad? Surely they are different, since there are things that Alan would have given them that I cannot.

I learned to accept that while I cannot be everything all the time, I can be enough, most of the time. At the conference in Austria during the ODDYsee, I was surprised to overhear someone refer to me as being a real brick. Whereas I viewed myself as just hanging on in the ongoing white-knuckle sail, someone else saw me as strong, capable and in control. Yet, here I was a few years later, still worried about my children and their well-being, my career and the future. At certain times of the year, I seem to exist in a state of utter mayhem when my professional academic world meets my family world head-on – for paper presentations at conferences, exam marking at Christmas, required presentation days and teaching during the children's March break, and exam marking that coincides with birthday parties, not to mention the times when bones break, stomach flu hits, yet another pet bird (Sunny) flies out the door and never comes back, and, somehow the pipe in the wall below the kitchen sink gets plugged by mysterious and unknown forces. It helps to have a sense of humour through all of this. In one short period, I realized that being a brick was going to be an ongoing and essential feature of my life. As I approached the third anniversary of Alan's death, I sent this e-mail to a friend, after a particularly bizarre winter day when, clearly, I needed to share.

Subject: Laughing hysterically

Well it's been one of those days, so I'm going to off-load because, well, just because.

6:00 a.m. Dogs, who wouldn't go out last night because of cold, go out.

6:01 Dogs return to bed, sigh as they sink into the warmth and fail to notice me bug-eyed and alert; worrying about office issue begins.

7:00 Wash hair; no solution to office issue. Day starts in earnest, don't wanna get up x 3. Sarah showers (teens do a lot of that) and screeches when Andrew flushes (I think it was innocent, but I can never be sure).

7:30: Breakfast x 4, memo to self: milk running low – easy fix: get after consultation about Sarah's toe at children's hospital.

7:45: Andrew and Carolyn dropped off for before-school care. I am in control again.

8:00: Arrive at hospital for consultation on Sarah's ingrown toenail. Doctor tied up elsewhere. Sensing a distinct shift in the karma of the day, I buy a large double-double coffee.

8:10: Doctor arrives. Announces that Sarah's toe needs outpatient surgery. Offers now or Monday. (Monday no good for Sarah or for me; opt for now. Milk pickup now off schedule, but can do after meeting in afternoon.) Still in control of situation. I look forward to watching doctors do their work. Heck, I have a hot coffee, it's quiet and I'm sitting down – all good signs.

8:15: Doctor freezes toe. Sarah not impressed; leaves dents in my hands from squeezing. Takes three injections deep into toe.

8:30: Doctor and brand-new pediatric emergency rotation doctor remove strip of toenail and tissue from either side of toe plus remove growth centre below bottom edge of nail in the same zones. Both doctors clearly think I am a very strange bird, since I want to observe everything. I am allowed to do so, provided I remain seated at all times (parents faint, I gather).

10:00: After required waiting to observe bleeding, blood pressure, etc., Sarah is back home in my bed, watching my VCR with painkillers, etc. Dogs agree to go outside but return to my bed with Sarah in it with foot elevated and Tylenol chaser every four hours.

11:00: Having answered office e-mail, I head downtown for a meeting about straightforward issue. At briefing, we are told that it is no longer a straightforward issue. So much for milk pickup solution #2.

3:30: Meeting finishes; return to university for class.

4:00: Nice, straightforward lecture in hot room. Note students waving in warm breezes of my scintillating lecture, some have odd neck-snapping-back motions. End of lecture brings another office issue e-mail. Try again, while driving home, to determine date of earliest possible retirement. Determine that tomorrow is not it.

5:30: Blessed be the other mother who drove Andrew and Carolyn home from their after-school program. They were supposed to walk. Blessed be the staff who realized that a drive was better than a walk and used common sense about permission, since we often drive each other's kids home after work. (Note: guilt meter had been in the red zone because of the walk home on the coldest day of the year and their long day, 7:45 a.m. to 5:30 p.m., at school.)

6:00 p.m.: Arrive home to broken VCR (teen crisis), broken water main on street – large, freezing men are wandering the neighbourhood searching for source of water and break, and Sarah's toe is bleeding through the dressing (shouldn't be). Note visible line of blood on bandage and check every 30 minutes. Boyfriend 1.0 has dropped off homework (chaperoned by girlfriend, as is the rule). Toilets can't be flushed (no water). Low milk is now no milk. Dinner plans shot without water or milk.

6:05: Reinvent dinner – Kraft Dinner, microwave style, needs only 1.75 cups of water and eight minutes. Kettle had two cups of water. Can't wash salad; there goes the serving of veggies. Sarah lounges in my bedroom eating dinner and chatting to friends on MSN. At suggestion that she do dropped-off homework, toe starts to ache – coincidence, perhaps.

6:20: Carolyn leaves for Girl Guides. Blessed be another mother who was on for driving.

6:30: Sarah announces major science test next day. I suggest missing it – after all, she has medical permission. Sarah demonstrates damaged DNA of both parents and insists on going for major test. Mummy (P.Eng.) digs out crutches used by Dad (180 pounds, 6 feet) when he broke his leg sailing eighteen years earlier (before Sarah was even a twinkle) and cuts them down for teenage girl (100 pounds, 5 feet). VCR fix simple: clean heads.

7:40: Crutch tips no longer flexible after eighteen years in basement. I finally make trip to drugstore for milk and crutch tips, but settle for cane tips and wonder whether they will work. I remember myself on crutches at seventeen and cringe, hoping own child will have more brains than to race male friend down hallway (I won, by the way). Perhaps non-racing father's DNA will prevail.

8:30: Pick up Girl Guides. Fill car. Gas light is on and I sense bad luck is in the air today. Add Guide skate-a-thon and sleepover to schedule for next week.

9:00: Complete Grade 4 homework; make lunches; make mental note to self that I am probably laughing hysterically at inane television show, since Sarah does not seem to think it is at all funny.

9:30: Calm begins as Grade 4s go to bed. Waterline of blood on toe dressing stabilizes. Toe appears to have stopped bleeding, meaning that I do not have to find a late-night sitter and go to emergency room. Pour myself medicinal sherry now that I don't have to drive or appear as calm rational parent.

10:00: Want hot bath; no can do – no water. Try e-mail therapy instead. Sleep tight.

Moyra

Within a day or two, I had wandered into a travel agency and picked up all kinds of brochures. Brick or no brick, I needed a break! It was time for a brief escape from reality.

Alan was still very much a part of our lives, and we often talked about what he would have said or done when certain things happened. After chaos had invaded our lives through events such as those described in my e-mail above, or when it was dark, snowy, cold or raining, Alan would usually mutter something about life being a real pain and then buy a lottery ticket and start planning our next camping trip, naturally scheduled to occur in the warm weather and sun. The children and I looked over the brochures and, since we had enjoyed our getaway cruise with him so much, we decided to take another on the upcoming

Easter weekend. On this trip, the kids were old enough that I could actually relax a bit. On one occasion, they all went back to the cabin to watch a movie and I stayed and finished a leisurely dinner in the dining room. At the first beach, the children instinctively made dribble sandcastles. Alan would have been delighted. It was an enjoyable hiatus from the blustery winds of chaos in my life.

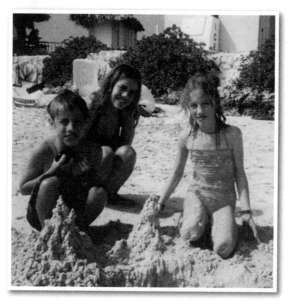

ANDREW, SARAH AND CAROLYN AND THE INEVITABLE DRIBBLE CASTLES, BAHAMAS.

Chaos was so normal that early one morning, before an important meeting, I found myself rushing with sopping hair and wearing high heels and a business suit to the animal hospital with Sweety the lovebird. After a night of labour she was unable to deliver her latest egg and died in intensive care – complete with a saline IV and on oxygen. Her vet bill was four times her original cost. Some months later, her lovebird pal Plucky somehow strangled himself on a small thread in the cage. Our small animal graveyard was becoming overly full.

It's hard sometimes, going through the daily motions of life with all its challenges, to make room for spontaneous silliness. I became more determined to make space for fun within the constraints of work and school. Fun can be something as simple as dropping everything and driving to the lake for a swim, renting a movie and staying up really late to watch it, having a picnic in the backyard, buying lots of fireworks for Canada Day, going on a fall hike that ends with a night in a tent, even when it's miserable, cold and raining, or taking a canoe trip with friends in the spring. I began to realize that it was time to invest more in making life happen. I intuitively felt that I was now on the path to somewhere new; I just had no idea where it was!

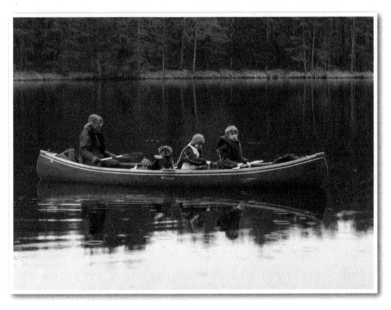

MOYRA, PENNY IN HER RAINCOAT, CAROLYN,
SCOOTER AND ANDREW IN ALGONQUIN PARK.

Through the Open Door

When a friend asked whether I still missed Alan, I was able to say that I would always miss him and I would always love him, but that the awful ache was now gone. The big emptiness that formed when he died has been, for the most part, filled again, although from time to time I still feel lonely. As I have made big decisions alone, things such as choosing schools for the children, putting a new roof on the house and buying a new van, the nighttime loneliness has subsided. I have become more comfortable being my own adviser but that doesn't mean everything is perfect. Sometimes I am still afraid of all the what-ifs that are out there. The biggest what-if is simple. What if I get sick? Then what? So, while I see my doctor for a physical and get my flu shot and try to stay fit, I know there are no guarantees. My children also know, all too well, that there are no guarantees. All I can do is make sure there are backup plans in place, that the children know what those plans are, and hope that they won't be needed. Certainly, the first few times a virus knocked me down for a few days, I could tell the children were worried, so we discussed what might happen if I did get sick – who would make decisions if I could not and who would be in charge if I died. We also agreed that I would be an organ donor. If my organs, like their dad's corneas, could be used to improve or save a life, so much the better.

Every morning, I imagine myself loading into my life the things that matter most to me: the children, the dogs, my career in engineering that supports us, and my mother, whose needs are steadily increasing. Life is fantastically busy and chaos is still a regular feature of it. I can find myself icing a birthday cake after midnight and buying birthday presents the morning of or even the week after the birthday in question. While I can't say that I embrace the chaos, I've learned that for me, and for now, it's a given. Shoving one more thing into our lives can usually work. So when my mother had hip replacement surgery and subsequent rehabilitation, it was natural that her cat, Little One, should come to live with our dogs, Scooter and Penny, and our latest lovebirds, Giblets (he appeared to wish to become giblets) and Oly (named for the 2004 Olympics). There was one proviso: the birds were not allowed to fly freely about the house.

It was natural that we should feel comfortable taking another little life into our home. Once home, this half-wild puss was immediately adopted by Carolyn, who had him purring and kneading and sleeping with her in a matter of days. The dogs tolerated the cat, provided he remained off the floor. In turn, the cat snuck about the house at night when the dogs were sleeping. Little One would often be found in the morning sitting on a dining room chair, admiring the antics of the caged birds. His arrival on the scene added some excitement but the dogs agreed that the Christmas spirit of peace on earth could be observed, at least long enough to take this picture.

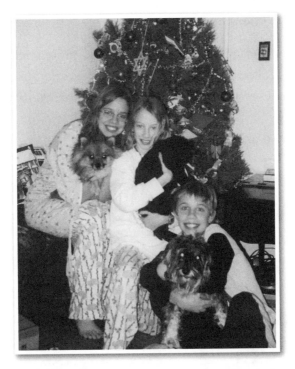

SARAH HOLDING SCOOTER, CAROLYN HOLDING LITTLE ONE,
AND ANDREW HOLDING PENNY, CHRISTMAS MORNING.

When my father-in-law passed away very close to the fourth anniversary of Alan's death. I revisited many of the emotions I had when Alan died. My own dad had died, when Sarah was a tiny baby, after a long fight with Alzheimer's, and Alan's dad had become a second father to me. Simply knowing he was out there had been a comfort. He had been very helpful at those times when Alan was feeling at odds with everything – in particular, when he was at odds with me. Perhaps there is in each of us a tiny piece that still listens to our parents, even when we can't or won't listen to our spouse.

Once again, we were all reminded of the circle of life. It was not a welcome visitor, but it was one we had met before. We reread *Water Bugs and Dragonflies* and talked about the happy times of family reunions and family dinners, and especially the memories we have of Alan and his dad sailing together.

I marked this passage in our lives by taking Andrew and Carolyn on an overnight canoe trip with friends from the office. Since Sarah was off at another event in her own busy life, we learned that the three of us can manage, and that marked another kind of passage. Of course, the dogs joined us for the adventure.

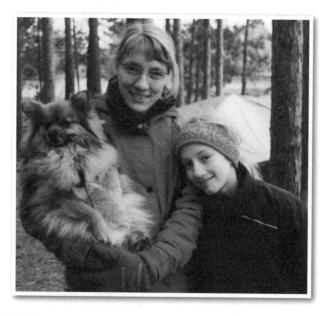

SCOOTER, MOYRA AND CAROLYN ON A CHILLY OVERNIGHT CANOE TRIP.

In the late spring, I helped Sarah and a few other girls from her high school track team learn to hurdle. There I stood on a track that was modern before even I was a high school athlete, trying to explain to

Sarah how to do three steps between the hurdles. Clearly it needed to be demonstrated, and so I did. It had been 30 years since I last hurdled. I had regained the courage (or perhaps the stupidity) to run full speed at fences. It wasn't pretty, but it did the trick. The next day I was stiff in places that I had forgotten I had, but I had regained something I thought was lost forever. It felt great. I smiled for several days. Deep inside, a change had taken place. Perhaps since I could once again face running at physical fences, I could tackle some of life's more challenging fences as well. It felt a bit like a new beginning.

I had read the letters Alan had written to our children when I read his letter to me. Although the letters were gentle and loving, I had decided to wait until the children were older to give them their letters. I gave Sarah hers on her sixteenth birthday. It took her several days to find the courage to open it. The message is mixed but, above all, is that of a daddy who loved his first little girl so very, very much. I think it is significant that she offered to include it in this book in the first week of Advent nearly five months later – a new beginning for her, too, perhaps.

> *To my darling Sarah,*
>
> *As I write this, you are just about to become a young lady. The years we have had together have been far too short. You may not know how proud your mum and I are about how you've turned out. You are a bright, clever girl who works hard at everything she does. More importantly, you are a nice person. We have been proudest of the way you help out at school or with others in your class. Don't ever change that. I hardly know what to say that would be good advice to you in your years to come. I suspect there is nothing that you wouldn't be smart enough to do anyway. The best thing I can think of is to recommend following your mum's advice. She is the smartest person I ever met.*
>
> *I am writing this at a time when you have really only recently outgrown being a little girl. I think I have probably been harder on you than the other two, which is something I regret. I have not decided what age you should receive this. High school seems too late. Shortly after I have*

died might be best, if that is what must happen. Any older and you'll be too certain of yourself to listen much. I know I was. This will be a mixed message: be humble but be confident. You have talents you haven't even thought of yet. Some you know; some you will find out as time goes by. Be patient. Life is a long journey, not a race. Get a good education. Things that really matter take years to build. Let life unfold easily and don't try to force things. I was never patient enough. I don't know how patient you are or will be.

Don't be too frightened of other people. Mostly they are lonely and scared. Some might try to humiliate you, but to hell with them. Be honest and pleasant. It really never pays to needlessly make enemies or be deliberately hurtful. If some are unpleasant back to you, then you really don't want to know them anyway. There are bad people out there, so do be careful. Mostly, however, they are not worth the aggravation – better to learn which ones they are sooner than later. Unfortunately, most men are selfish swine, so do be careful. I'd look to the shy and quiet ones who would, I hope, have a better appreciation for someone as special as you and know how lucky they are to be a friend of yours.

One enduring characteristic of our family has been its lack of self-confidence. With more talent than any ten average people, we still contrive to sell ourselves short. One thing I have learned is that normal people are not nearly so clever or devious as we give them credit for. All human activities, from plumbing to rocket science, are done by people who are by definition mostly unskilled and not very intelligent.

I love all you guys, in spite of how it may appear from my behaviour. It brings tears to my eyes when I think of what I'll be missing or have missed. Whatever happens, do enjoy your lives together.

The time may come when I don't recognize you or forget your name. It doesn't mean that I've stopped loving you, only that the cancer has eaten that part of my brain, not that part of my heart.

I doubt if there is anything much that needs changing in you. First, don't worry too much about what others think or see in you. It's important to get along with people and not be unpleasant, but remember, most of them are as frightened as you are and struggling as best they can to get by.

Mostly, they are busy trying to hide their own faults to be able to see much that you may have done wrong. Don't be too negative about yourself and your accomplishments. People are not critically watching you, waiting for a mistake. Don't be lazy; work hard but try to not let work and career become a total focus. Hard work and talent are what matter. You have the second and can control the first. Be sure to enjoy your life.

Take lessons in self-defence and get very good at them.

If you have trouble with depression then, for goodness sake, don't wait as long as I did before getting treatment. This, more than anything else, has probably blighted my career, wasted years of my life and hurt my family, all because I was too stubborn to admit I might need help. I must have wasted fifteen years of my life. It's no sin to admit that you might need help. It doesn't lessen anything but improves the bonds between friends and colleagues.

Life is about making choices and balancing the consequences of those choices. Choosing between the shorter-term fun and the longer-term benefits is a constant problem. I think I may have focused on the longer-term results a bit much, but however one balances things, whatever the results are, it is possible to look back and wonder whether the other choice would have been better. Most of all, take care to have some fun along the way. One thing I do know is that life is shorter than you think. Enjoy what you have while it's here and try more new things, even if you are bad at them. It's a mark of courage to try, even if you look bad, than to not try at all. Besides, you learn something even when things don't work out. New skills and new knowledge are always valuable.

When encountering life's problems, be a cork, not a stone. The cork will ride out the problems bobbing on the waves, while the stone sinks to the bottom. I spent too much time being a rock, trying to force the waves to break around me. It doesn't work that way.

Finally, reputations are built on successes. Don't worry too much about making mistakes. Try not to make too many mistakes but don't let the fear of making a mistake paralyze you into doing nothing. Mostly, nobody cares except you when you make the odd mistake.

Most of all, I love you and your brother and sister and mother. What I'll miss most of all is not being with all of you to see you growing up.

Alan

How far we had come since Alan wrote his letters to the children. They were indeed growing up, and I would soon learn just how much. Several years earlier, when I had been part of the organizing committee for the 12th International Conference of Women Engineers and Scientists, I promised the children I would take them to the next one, which was to be held in Seoul, South Korea, in 2005. I presented two papers, one technical and one related to women in engineering, both co-authored with students. After the conference, we went to Jeju Island for a short tour. The entire trip was an introduction to another language and culture. We swam in the Pacific Ocean, saw Hwa Seong fortress, ate very different food than we were used to, slept ondol style on a heated floor, and encountered Korean schoolchildren on their own school trips. It was a fantastic adventure.

Coincidentally, the conference overlapped the seventh anniversary of Alan's diagnosis and what would have been our 27th wedding anniversary. As I walked around the walls of Hwa Seong fortress and later along the volcanic rocky shore of Jeju Island, I thought of how much Alan would have enjoyed being there. Alan loved to travel. He was particularly fond of castles and, of course, he was drawn to the ocean.

Naturally, my thoughts went back over the years and especially to those days when my four-year-old twins and nine-year-old daughter sat on the side of their daddy's hospital bed. I had been so worried then that Alan's influence would be lost with time and that I might not be able to raise them all on my own. Now, I could see how they had grown. I could see their strength, their courage, their confidence, their excitement. I could see very welcome traces of their dad in them: their collective openness to seeing the world; Andrew's curiosity, which led him to climb up and peer over a fortress wall; Carolyn's willingness to try exotic foods, including eating raw sea snail and raw sea squirt just pulled from the ocean floor; and Sarah's enthusiastic interaction with the adult world, drinking it all in and always carrying a book to read in those quiet moments, just as Alan had done.

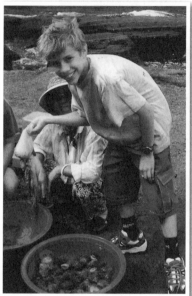 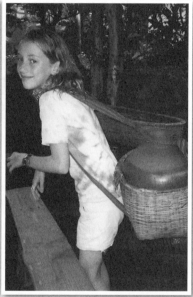

ANDREW HOLDS AN OCTOPUS TAKEN FROM THE OCEAN BY A FEMALE FREE DIVER, AND CAROLYN CARRIES A TRADITIONAL WATER BOTTLE, ON JEJU ISLAND.

On the last full day of our trip, I sat quietly on a small beach, watching the children swim in the Pacific, play in the sand and explore the rocky shore. I was aware of a sense of deep contentment – something I hadn't felt for a long time. Then, as improbable as it sounds, a Canadian colleague began to play Celtic music on her fiddle. The dichotomy was startling. Something from my distant heritage was being played on a beach in South Korea! My past met my present and I found myself looking into my future along that continuum of experience that stretches from generation to generation. I am a product of everything I have encountered. Alan and the love we shared will always be part of me, and our children will carry him into their futures. I can look to those little fragments of experience to reassure me and make sense of things. I had reached a kind of inner peace with the entire experience. It was time to make the final entry in my logbook and close its cover.

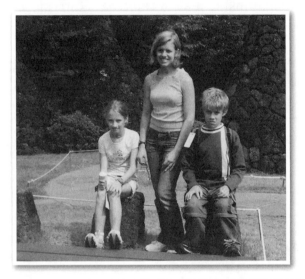

CAROLYN, SARAH AND ANDREW AT A TEA PLANTATION ON JEJU ISLAND.

There is joy to be found in investing in life and all of its experiences. There is pleasure in the companionship of our pets. We can chuckle as the porcupines fearlessly lumber along the lake road in front of the car. We can smile with delight as the ducklings fledge each year, marking the passage of time, and when a hawk flies over the lake, we can remember Alan.

I have walked through the open door to a precious, chaotic, hectic and unpredictable life that continues to unfold around me.

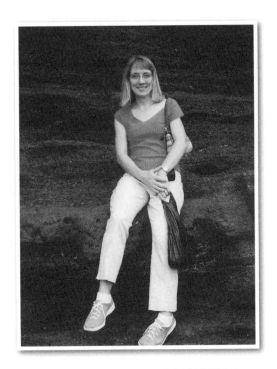

MOYRA LOOKS OUT OVER THE PACIFIC OCEAN.